Stop Painful Sex: Healing from Vaginismus. A Step-by-Step Guide

Maree Stachel-Williamson

ISBN-13: 978-1505255157
ISBN-10: 1505255155

CONTENTS

ACKNOWLEDGMENTS

Thank you to Leigh for giving me an insight into the experience from your point of view and giving your blessing on sharing our experiences in this book.

Thank you to Janaya. Back then I think you were the only other person I felt I could confide in about this topic. Thank you for being there for me.

Thank you to my clinical supervisor Ruby who told me to "go for it".

Thank you to my colleague and friend Laurinda-Lee for helping me realize just how important it was that I got this information out there and for including my personal story. I also appreciate the time you gave with your eagle eyes to notice my many spelling and grammatical mistakes.

And thank you to my understanding and loving husband Jan for all his hours listening and helping me with this project – especially with all the final editing work. Thank you for also encouraging me to take the first steps in becoming a therapist. And a huge thank you for your support, understanding and wisdom as I have worked through my issues over the years.

1. INTRODUCTION

My story and why I have written this book for you.

I used to suffer from vaginismus. And when I say suffer, I mean suffer. Sex was incredibly painful. Even worse, sexual intercourse was physically impossible.

When I had vaginismus I didn't know such a thing even existed. It was the late 1990's. I was 17 years old and experienced it for nearly a year. I never spoke to a doctor or health professional about it and it wasn't until several years ago when I started getting referrals from a sexual health clinic for NLP (Neuro Linguistic Programming) and hypnotherapy to help women who were experiencing painful sex. I was asked to teach the women referred to me how to relax, help them understand the role of the unconscious mind and work through any related traumas. It was then that I consciously realized I had suffered from the same condition in my youth. It was an incredible moment because it felt as though, for the first time in my life, what I had been through became something that officially 'existed'.

The female clients being referred to me are sometimes embarrassed and confused about the situation. Given that there is no external funding for appointments, they often come in for a chat or a session after being recommended to do so by the clinic. Sometimes they are still trying to get their head around what is actually happening and unsure about what they want to do to try to solve it (or whether it can be solved in the first place).

So in the little time I see them, I might get the chance to talk to them about the role of the unconscious mind, and teach them some relaxation exercises. When appropriate, I can help them work through the memory of a traumatic sexual experience. We may explore the bigger picture and the current issues in their relationship. But there is never enough time to do all (or even a quarter) of that which would be useful. Often I have wished I could tell them about a really useful self-help program or book. Ideally it would be a kind of informative workbook that would help them learn and explore all aspects of the situation. The kind of book that would not only inform, but also one that is packed with practical steps so they could pinpoint the source of the issue for them personally and start to do something about it – in their own time and pace, in privacy and with little cost involved.

The more I thought about this, the more obvious it became that I needed to create that book for them (and for all the others, like me, who do not even seek help in the first place). The fact that I have had vaginismus myself means that I could incorporate elements and insights from a personal level as well as the knowledge I have gained as a therapist.

Personally, I've always been into dreaming big and in my healing from vaginismus, it was important to me to not only be able to have sexual intercourse, but to have mind blowing, beautiful, spiritual sexual experiences and be able to experience all that my body was capable of experiencing. I have had this in mind as I have written this book. It is not just about stopping the pain, but working towards a strong emotional connection and really enjoyable sex with whoever you may choose.

Because there can often be a lot to overcome in terms of psychological hurdles for a woman with vaginismus, I believe it is important to look not just at getting over the emotional blocks and fears but also to work towards body acceptance and responsibility for one's own pleasure. Knowing your body and being able to control your own arousal is an empowering position to be in which will benefit sexual and intimate relationships well into the future.

Therefore in this book, I not only look at helping you understand the condition of vaginismus and how it is that you may have come to have it as well as steps you can take to overcome it, but I also approach the larger topic of sexual enjoyment and masturbation. Of course whether you want to explore masturbation is entirely up to you. It's an experience I highly recommend because just as it is important to know how to make yourself happy rather than having to wait for someone else to 'give' you happiness, it also makes sense and is most empowering to be able to pleasure yourself and reap the benefits – emotionally, physically and spiritually, without having to pin your needs on someone else being able to fulfill them for you. In my eyes masturbation is the ultimate form of sexual freedom. Women are more likely to orgasm during sex in a long term relationship than from casual sex, and thus taking responsibility and learning how to give yourself this pleasure just makes logical sense so you can experience it regardless of your situation.

So there I was as a teenager when I became sexually active with my first long-term boyfriend. I remember consciously choosing to lose my virginity with him even though we weren't officially going out at the time. For ease of reading, I will simply refer to him in this book as my first boyfriend. I felt physically very safe with him and since our past sexual experiences had been very pleasurable I assumed making love would be as well. Being educated at a Catholic school had planted some negative thoughts and fears in my mind and I really wanted my first time to be a positive memory. Much to my horror, what followed was months of trying again and again to lose my virginity. No matter what we did, it was always painful for me. My body didn't seem as if it was going to allow me to lose my virginity. If you suffer from vaginismus, you know what I'm talking about.

The way I remember it is that he would have a very difficult time 'getting in', and would thrust a little but I'd be in tears and ask him to stop. We would pause and then try again hoping the pain would just stop if we kept going, but it never did and we would always have to give up. Interestingly, I later discovered that he remembered as not being able to enter me at all – in his words, it was as though he was hitting a wall. It was exhausting for both of us – emotionally and physically.

He ended up dealing with feelings of inadequacy and frustration and I feared even more that he must surely be cheating on me. I realize that technically he couldn't 'cheat' as we weren't officially together, but I nonetheless felt as though we were due to our intimacy. He already had quite a reputation, so my trust in his being faithful during this time was pretty fragile which lead to additional fear of catching a sexually transmitted disease and generally feeling used. Of course being teenagers, neither of us thought to talk about it or to let each other know what we were thinking. Looking back, neither of us had the skills and confidence to broach the topic in a useful way.

Having this experience wore away at us and almost took away all the fun of being intimate because this was always looming in our minds before we had even started. Eventually we went our separate ways again.

Some time after a short-lived relationship that ended before it became sexual, I started dating again and when I 'risked' attempting sexual intercourse with my new partner I was surprised to discover the vaginismus had completely gone. There was no pain at all, not even a hint of difficulty.

When I think back to the time when I had vaginismus, my heart goes out to my younger self. It was such a difficult thing to go through on top of all the other teenage ups and downs that were already stressful enough. I wish I had had a book like this back then that described to me in simple English what was happening to me, why it was happening and how I could take the matter into my own hands and get rid of it earlier.

It didn't occur to us to seek professional help. Even if I had thought of it, I'm pretty sure I would have been too embarrassed to do so anyway. Getting the kind of information that is in this book would have been extremely useful for both myself and my first boyfriend at the time. We could have avoided all the confusion, horrible feelings, pain and loss of self-confidence.

How to use this book

Throughout this book I have tried to use as little jargon as possible, be it medical or technical, to make it easy to understand and follow. I have instead used my own words and simple descriptions as much as possible.

There might be sections in this book that you are already knowledgeable about and bits you might find boring. Feel free to skip from one section to the next as it suits you.

This book includes an integrated workbook. Aside from physical exercises, it includes questions which help by guiding you in the exploration and discovery of your beliefs, thoughts and feelings about sex and sexuality. I have found this self-discovery process a vital part in my own journey (which continued long after the symptoms disappeared) as it helped me understand why I thought or felt a certain way. Sometimes just by finding out this information I've felt free to choose a new way of thinking as I realized the belief or emotion originated from somewhere or someone else. You might like to use a special note book or journal where you can write down your thoughts and reactions to the questions and exercises. Workbook questions are indicated in *italics* throughout the book. Other questions, mainly the post couple exercise ones aren't necessarily labeled as workbook questions because I want you to discuss your experience together with your partner. However, of course following it up with reflection in your journal may be useful as well.

I have included a lot of exercises and I want to urge you to only do those you feel comfortable doing. Complete them at your own pace and feel free to explore one particular exercise over a period of time. There is no rule that says you need to take this journey in any specific way. It's your life, your body and your choice. So find a way that works for you.

Disclaimer

I'm a female in a long-term marriage with a history of heterosexual mostly long-term relationships. Throughout the writing of this book, I have found myself naturally speaking from my point of view and personal experience. However, I am aware that some of the readers of this book may be lesbian or bisexual. And in addition, some may not be in a long-term relationship.

So please forgive me if I talk of sexual intercourse occurring with a vagina and penis or if I refer to a partner or boyfriend. I do not mean to offend and for every situation I write about there are of course other ways and techniques that do not require a male nor a penis. Sometimes I have included comments to address that, other times I am sure I have forgotten. Please bear with me in those moments and accept my apologies.

This book is not meant to replace therapy but to complement it. The exercises in this book are provided as self-exploration techniques, some which you can do by yourself and some with a partner. Depending on your situation and the reasons why you are experiencing vaginismus, there may be some exercises that are emotionally challenging. For example, if you have been sexually abused you may find extreme emotions come up and for that reason I strongly recommend that you start sessions with an experienced therapist who can provide support for you. It might be best to start sessions with your therapist before trying out any of the exercises in this book.

Throughout this book I regularly recommend having additional support from health professionals including a therapist. That is because, ideally, if you have been experiencing vaginismus for a while, I believe getting additional support would be useful. I do however acknowledge from my own and others' situations that this is sometimes not desired or accessible at least not initially. If this is the case for you then I hope that you make good progress with this book, find alternative supports within your network of family and friends and read as many books, blogs and websites about this as you can.

Some of the content of this book may also stretch your beliefs or challenge your comfort zone and I'm not doing this to offend you! I've included everything in this book so that you can get the best learning experience out of reading it and to clearly describe the condition and what you can do about it.

Please make sure that you are well supported emotionally while reading this book, to make your journey as comfortable as possible. Support could also come from a close friend, your partner or a trusted family member.

So let's start.

2. PART ONE: THE BIOLOGY AND PSYCHOLOGY OF VAGINISMUS

What is vaginismus?

First of all, what is vaginismus? Here is a definition of what it is and what it is not, to make it easier for you to understand what is actually going on down there.

Vaginismus is the term used for vaginal pain caused specifically by the muscles in the outer third of the vagina involuntarily contracting during or in anticipation of penetration. The result is that penetration is either difficult and painful or impossible due to the vaginal muscles contracting to such an extent that any attempt at entry feels like 'hitting a wall'. Vaginismus is not a choice and some women (including me) might not even be aware of the muscles tensing when it happens. In addition, and not surprisingly, the condition typically causes emotional distress and difficulty within the sexual relationship.

For the purposes of being able to understand your personal experience it can be useful to recognize the specifics of what you have been experiencing, because there are different types of vaginismus:

Lifelong – For some, the pain begins upon the first attempt of vaginal penetration and can last a lifetime, especially if not addressed in therapy or with your doctor. Vaginismus is the number one reason behind unconsummated marriages.

Acquired – For others it occurs after a period of time. The woman experiences normal functioning and then vaginismus appears – sometimes suddenly. Examples of this could be pain occurring after an experience of having sexual intercourse while emotionally distressed or after a physical condition has caused an experience of painful sex.

General – Another differentiation is sometimes made in the medical world when it appears as a general reaction whenever any vaginal penetration is attempted (including the attempted use of tampons).

Situational – This type of vaginismus is when the symptoms only happen in specific situations such as with a particular sexual partner or during a gynecological examination or specifically during sexual intercourse only whereas other penetrations are fine.

It is because of these differences in individuals' experience of vaginismus that I often refer to penetration rather than sexual intercourse.

You may have also come across the more general term 'dyspareunia' which is used to describe all types of sexual pain including after intercourse. Vaginismus in contrast is the term for the specific experience of the vaginal muscles tightening.

Basically, you can still have vaginismus despite being in otherwise good health, in a loving relationship in which you feel safe and otherwise enjoy sexual intimacy.

If you visit a medical professional to be diagnosed it is useful to be aware that, for diagnostic purposes, the two conditions vaginismus and dyspareunia have recently been combined because they often occur together and it's sometimes difficult for doctors to distinguish between the two. The new term in the latest DSM-5 the American Psychiatric Association's Diagnostic and Statistical Manual of Mental Disorders is 'Genito-Pelvic Pain/Penetration Disorder'.

Possible causes

To be diagnosed with this condition according to the DSM manual, there have to be psychological factors contributing to your experience rather than just medical causes. The following are some possible causes or contributing factors, however having had one or more of these experiences alone does not necessarily lead to vaginismus.

– **Childhood upbringing:** Being brought up in a strict religious setting with negative beliefs and teachings about sex and sexuality being passed down. These beliefs and teachings might have been clearly and openly communicated, e.g. being told "Don't touch yourself there or you will go to hell" or a negative view might have been hinted at, such as "You must remain pure and clean".

Workbook questions:
What names have you given your vagina over time?
What names did other people around you use for the vagina?
What do these names symbolize or imply? (E.g. just another part of the body, an area that is cute, dirty, silly, an area to be disrespected or abused or be ashamed of?)
How and what did you learn about sex, pleasure and your genitals as you were growing up?

– **Life experiences and messages** that might have contributed to any discomfort with sex and sexuality. Being given messages while growing up (overtly and covertly) that your genitals and anything to do with them is dirty or wrong or 'only for going to the toilet'. This includes being smacked or given a 'punishing look' for expressing your sexuality.

Workbook questions:
What did you learn directly or indirectly about sex and sexuality from:
Your Mother:
Your Father:
Your siblings:
Your friends:
Other family members:
Society:
Do you remember other sex related messages – for example, being told off for 'making love to your food'?

– **Fear, anxiety and expectation** that the first time having sex will be painful. Just as some people developed a phobia of sharks after watching the movie Jaws in the 1980s, women can develop a fear of the pain of sex from either what they have been told or from TV and other media. In addition, the imagination can intensify and strengthen the thought patterns and related emotions.

– When a woman experiences fear and anxiety during moments of intimacy, this can also lead to vaginal dryness and muscle tension.

– First time experiences can cause future expectations of pain: Lack of sufficient arousal and lubrication (when losing your virginity) can lead to a higher than otherwise level of pain.

– **Small tears in the sensitive skin tissue** around the entrance to the vagina or hymen or hymenal remnants (especially relevant for first time experiences) resulting from penetration while not being adequately lubricated or relaxed enough may lead to inflammation and nerve sensitization. However, it is useful to note that skin tissue in this area generally heals well and quickly.

– **Sexual abuse or rape**. Having an experience where your body is violated or someone has been intimate with you without your consent can create numerous emotional and physical reactions. These can include an involuntary contraction of the vaginal muscles during future sexual experiences even when these experiences are wanted.

– **High pelvic floor muscle tone**. Some studies indicate that having a naturally high pelvic floor muscle tone can be the cause of vaginismus (the PC muscle group – short for pubococcygeus – are the muscles surrounding the vagina and anus). In this case, the muscle is naturally tensed or at least partially contracted even while the person is resting and not being touched. It can be the case that women with a naturally high PC muscle tone clench this muscle when stressed in the same way that others might clench their jaws, shoulders or faces.

– **Underlying emotional issues or conflict**. Vaginismus can occur spontaneously in a relationship as an unconscious response when a women somehow feels uncomfortable in the relationship.

– **Menopause**. Entering and during menopause, it is common for a woman to start producing less vaginal fluid and feel drier than in her youth. Around this time, sex can become painful due to this dryness and if a woman persists despite the pain, this can also lead to vaginismus as her body starts reacting in the fear/anxiety response of tensing the vaginal muscles.

– **Other physical and medical situations**. There is a surprisingly high number of medical situations that can contribute to vaginismus due to them causing pain upon penetration. These include post childbirth, medications, starting and persisting with sexual intercourse despite inadequate vaginal lubrication, infections, sexually transmitted diseases, skin conditions such as eczema, vaginal prolapse, cysts or tumors, endometriosis, urinary tract infections and tipped uterus.

As I mentioned above, officially the diagnoses of vaginismus requires the presence of psychological factors contributing to your experience rather than just medical causes. However, it is understandable that having a number of or even a one-off negative experience of painful penetration can plant the seed of emotional discomfort and fear for future attempts.

Workbook questions:
What is your experience of vaginismus?
When does it happen? (Inserting a tampon? A finger? A specific situation only?)
When doesn't it happen?
When did it first start?
Which of the above possible causes relates to you and your life?

Understanding vaginismus – What's actually happening? The mind and body connection

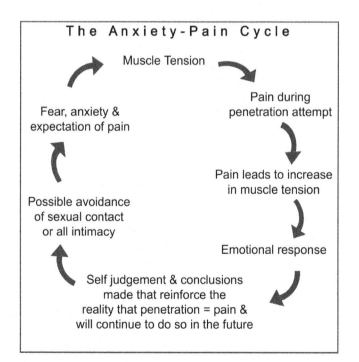

The Anxiety-Pain Cycle

Muscle Tension

Pain during penetration attempt

Fear, anxiety & expectation of pain

Pain leads to increase in muscle tension

Possible avoidance of sexual contact or all intimacy

Emotional response

Self judgement & conclusions made that reinforce the reality that penetration = pain & will continue to do so in the future

Due to the fact that vaginismus is not consciously chosen, created or desired, it is generally very confusing and a frustrating experience. It is often an unconsciously learned behavior which also continues to operate unconsciously.

Are you familiar with the idea of something happening 'unconsciously'? Sometimes people use the term subconscious rather than unconscious. Others use the two terms interchangeably. They mean the same thing in relation to what I'm talking about in this book. For those of you who are not familiar with these words, I'll try to explain it in a simple and easily understandable way.

When I refer to something happening unconsciously, I am not talking about when people are unconscious (in the medical sense), but rather mentally unaware. When we do something unconsciously, we do it without our conscious attention or awareness. For example, think about a skill you have. When you first started learning this skill, you were aware of all the steps you needed to take in order to get the results you wanted. You were still doing it consciously. Take riding a bike for example. I remember learning how to ride a bike with my father. I was very aware of the need to adjust my balance from side to side as I pedaled, making sure that I didn't topple off by leaning too much to one side as each foot pushed down or raised up. Actually I did topple and fall off a lot, but that's just part of learning isn't it. You could say, at that stage, I was consciously riding my bike.

Over time, as I mastered keeping my balance while riding, I could just sit back and ride. My thoughts were free to wander and focus on other things like noticing the traffic or the weather or a friend ahead of me. My conscious mind was free again for whatever I wanted to focus on. And the bike riding itself had become an unconscious behavior. Does that make sense?

Think about some activities you do that are unconscious. For example, if you drive somewhere, you might have certain regular routes you take that you drive unconsciously, not having to put any attention on which turns you have to take or where to go. Walking is something that for the majority of us is an unconscious behavior. Watch a baby learning to walk (or even stand) and then you realize how unconscious that behavior has become for you.

Similar to driving, walking or riding a bike, vaginismus is also an unconscious behavior. It's not a conscious choice. We don't consciously choose to tighten the muscles. It's like breathing. Most of the time we just do that automatically (unconsciously) as well.

What's happening is that the mind (unconsciously) is fearful or does not want to experience a situation (in this case pain upon penetration). Sometimes women with vaginismus aren't even aware that their unconscious mind has this fear.

Because of these feelings of fear or anxiety, breathing becomes shallow and the muscles automatically tighten. These anxious thoughts in combination with the shallow breathing may also release chemicals in the brain such as cortisol and adrenalin which in turn increases the fear response even more. So when penetration is attempted, the mind gets the feedback from the body (this is called biofeedback) that it was correct in its fear that it would be uncomfortable, because now it is!

This in turn leads to even more tightening of the muscles

as a self-protection mechanism, which leads to more pain or impossibility of penetration. You might stop, but then the anxiety will remain until next time, although now it is strengthened and justified through your experience. Thus at the following attempt the experience happens again. And again and again, unless the underlying unconscious concerns are addressed. What a frustrating situation!

The great news is that we can change unconscious behaviors including vaginismus. Just as you can learn a new breathing style by choosing to consciously focus on your breath and teaching yourself a new way to breathe, you can also focus on your muscles including the ones that cause vaginismus and teach yourself to relax instead. I'll be showing you how to do both later in this book.

3. SEX - DON'T GIVE UP ... IT'S GOOD FOR YOU! PHYSICAL AND EMOTIONAL BENEFITS FROM SEX

Some women give up trying to have sexual intercourse because of the physical and emotional pain that becomes associated with it. In my case, my fixation on not being able to have what I thought of as 'real' sex with my first boyfriend stopped me from fully relaxing and enjoying the pleasure I could still have.

So what's the big deal, right? If sex is painful, why bother trying? There are plenty of more important things to experience in life and in your relationship, right? Wrong! Well, you can be the judge, but aside from the abundant, free source of joy and pleasure that can be gained, there are some important reasons why learning to relax and enjoy the experience of sex makes a lot of sense.

Less stress: There are many health benefits of enjoying sex, including a reduction in stress. Research into sexuality in the western world began mainly in the U.S. by Alfred Kinsey in the 1950's, who published his very controversial Kinsey reports. He found that having sex reduces feelings of anxiety, violence, hostility and stress. Sex also plays a role in creating a general sense of well-being.

Live longer: A woman's enjoyment of sex has also been associated with a longer life in a study at Duke University. Okay, so you don't get any points for just 'doing it', to get this benefit you have to enjoy it too!

Help keep your relationship alive: Having sex allows your partner to experience you in one of your most vulnerable states. Making love creates feelings of intimacy, closeness, caring and playfulness in unique ways that other activities cannot achieve. Making time for connecting in an intimate and loving way helps a relationship become and remain a strong bond of connectedness well into old age.

Pain relief: Those who know me, know that I am a fan of natural remedies and it turns out that vaginal stimulation (as opposed to clitoral only stimulation) provides substantial pain relief. Therefore if you really do have a headache (rather than just a faked one "Honey I'd love to but I can't because I have a headache") you should actually have sex because it will help ease your headache. Unless, of course, you prefer pain medication.

Get fit: During sex, depending on the positions and activity, your heart and breathing rates increase, you're moving and using the muscles in your arms, legs, butt, back and abdomen and all of these combine to burn calories, boost your metabolism, contribute to muscle growth and tone as well as improving your overall fitness level.

Natural antidepressant: Sex helps us feel happy due to it having a wonderful side effect – acting like an antidepressant in our bodies.

Estrogen increase: The female body releases higher levels of estrogen into the blood during sex. Benefits of estrogen include a healthy cardiovascular system, healthier cholesterol levels, increased bone density, and supple skin. In addition to that, estrogen helps keep vaginal tissues supple and protects against heart disease and osteoporosis.

Use it or lose it: Just like any muscle, with age a woman's vagina will atrophy and lose its elasticity if it is not penetrated for a long period of time. Of course, this may not be an issue for someone who is not interested in having penetrative sex of any nature in future, but if you are interested in that, then know that penetration (whether from a penis, vibrator or dildo) keeps your vaginal muscles healthy.

What is the goal here?

So now that you know that sex is really good for your health both mentally and physically, that it might increase how long you live and improve your mood, it can be important to also look at your personal motivation to have sex ... apart from just 'getting it on' of course. Because let's face it, learning how to have and enjoy sexual intercourse is about so much more than just reaching 'home base' even though we may not always be aware of our deeper reasons for wanting to have sex. The journey you will take is one of exploration and learning to enhance the experience of your natural sexuality, arousal and pleasure – treating vaginismus is hardly a chore when you think about it like that!

When I was unable to have sexual intercourse because of vaginismus, I just wanted the pain to stop so I could enjoy a sense of full connection with my boyfriend. I imagined that having 'real' sex would enable us to connect at an even deeper emotional and spiritual level. Knowing that this was my higher goal, a good question I could have asked myself back then is 'How else can I deepen our connection?'

Knowing what your higher goal is can be a useful path to creating a sense of satisfaction and contentment despite what might be happening between the sheets right now. What is your higher goal that you imagine you would achieve through getting rid of vaginismus? How else could you achieve that?

People can get so focused on sexual goals and what is not working that they miss opportunities for fun, new experiences and the chance to deepen their emotional connection. Even couples who are problem-free in their sex life find that sex can become very unsatisfying if it becomes monotonous or just about reaching a certain goal like an orgasm.

Touch for the sake of touch is also a valid reason for sexual intimacy with your partner as doing so causes the brain to release the hormone oxytocin, which makes us feel loved and secure and helps decrease feelings of stress and anxiety.

It is important that making love does not become goal

oriented but is rather an act of enjoyment. As a psychotherapist once asked a couple running out of steam in a 100 day challenge (in which they were supposed to have sex every day) "What defines sex?" It's a good question when you think about it. I mean, who said sex is only about penetration? Loosening up your ideas of what sex is or is not and just enjoying the moment, the intimacy and the exploration of each other's bodies is a very good place to start.

The same is absolutely true with self-pleasuring. You will have a much more enjoyable experience each time if you simply give in to exploring what feels nice for you and following that rather than trying to orgasm or do it a certain way.

4. UNDERSTANDING THE FEMALE SEXUAL AROUSAL PROCESS

Education is generally an important part of treatment programs aiming to heal vaginismus. That means it's important to learn and understand not just about vaginismus itself but also the female body and how its sexual arousal process works.

There are many reasons why it can be useful to know and understand the stages a female body goes through during sexual arousal, the main one of which in my opinion is to be able to recognize within yourself 'where you are up to' in the process as you explore your body's own response whether during self-pleasuring or being intimate with a partner.

There are five main phases in the female arousal process sometimes referred to as the 'human response cycle': desire phase, excitement phase, plateau phase, orgasmic phase and resolution phase.

Visually, the following diagram illustrates the intensity as it is felt in the body throughout the individual phases.

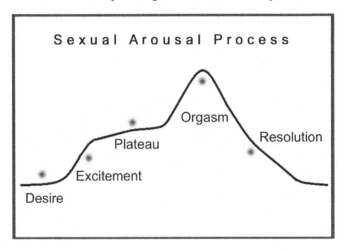

Desire phase

The desire phase in a woman's arousal can start when you are in some way stimulated. The stimulation could come via any of the senses – sight, touch, hearing, smell and taste. It is something that for you is erotically pleasing – whether part of a real situation such as seeing a naked body, reading erotic literature, sharing affection, tasting a romantic and delicious meal, or sexual fantasies in your mind, thoughts or memories that spark arousal and desire. For some women, desire for sexual contact might not be based on sexual desire but is based on a longing or need to connect emotionally with their partner and feel loved, accepted or emotionally close. In addition, some women might be waiting a long time before they have sex if they waited until they feel sexually aroused. Sometimes a woman will not get turned on until she is actually being touched in an intimate way. This has led some sex therapists to urge couples to initiate sex even if they aren't necessarily 'in the mood', because touch itself can trigger desire.

Workbook questions:
What sparks desire in you?
Physical triggers:
Visual triggers:
Olfactory triggers (smell):
Gustatory triggers (taste):
Acoustic triggers (sound):
Which is your biggest turn on out of the above?
What sparks desire for your partner? Do you know?
What are your fantasies?

Excitement phase

The excitement phase is the body's aroused response to the thoughts and feelings of desire. It is possible to start to get physically aroused without realizing it consciously or actually feeling mentally or emotionally aroused. In this phase, heart rate and blood pressure rise and there is an increase in muscular tension in the body. In light skinned women, there can be a noticeable flushing of the skin around the chest area. Nipples may become erect and as blood flow increases to body tissues, the clitoris, labia, and nipples swell and become darker. The vagina also starts to moisten as it secretes lubricating fluids. The length of this stage can vary according to amount and effectiveness of the stimulation. As they reach menopause, many women may find this initial phase takes longer with the body needing more stimulation before it releases enough lubrication for penetration.

Plateau phase

This is an extension of the excitement phase and a kind of leveling off before orgasm. If stimulation continues, the sexual tension increases and you more and more desire the release of the tension by having an orgasm. As arousal rises from the initial excitement phase, the vulva becomes more swollen and the clitoris, if it hasn't already, becomes more erect and exposed from the hooded skin around it. The area around the nipples, called the areola, also swells.

Some sexual practices such as Tantric Sex teach how to prolong this phase, which can lead to more intense orgasms and the ability to quickly become re-aroused and experience further orgasms. For many people, learning how to simply relax into and enjoy this phase can be a very rewarding experience whether as part of practicing how to be in the moment and allowing oneself to feel and reside in a state of pleasure. Or in the case of making love with a partner, it can be beneficial to enhance feelings of connection and emotional intimacy.

Orgasm phase

During orgasm, the uterus and lower third of the vagina contract in waves. In addition, you may also experience waves of contractions or jolts throughout your body. Each woman experiences a different intensity and length of orgasm. Also, you will find similarities and differences between your own orgasms. Research and studies show that the majority of woman reach this climactic phase through some kind of clitoral stimulation.

Resolution phase

After orgasm, the muscles start to relax and there a sense of overall relaxation. Heart rate and blood pressure decrease. Any flushing of the skin disappears and the engorged tissues in the labia and clitoris return to their normal state as do the nipples and areola. The clitoris also retreats back to its original position and can be extremely sensitive.

If stimulation is discontinued at this point then the body will return to its normal, unaroused state within around 30 minutes. If stimulation continues then you might go through the excitement and plateau phase again (often faster this time) and have another orgasm.

Some sexologists and sex therapists have argued that this model is too simple and unrealistic with its basic outline of the stages, and I agree. Here's why:

Firstly, there are some women who do not experience an orgasm. Sometimes this is because they have not experienced one before and sometimes women may not orgasm due to choice or otherwise. While some women naturally stumble across the experience of orgasms during their sexual exploration and experiences, others have to put in some effort and those who know how to sometimes may choose to simply focus on expressing love through touch and are satisfied by the intimacy itself.

In addition, sexual arousal is not a straightforward process and people can jump from one phase to another such as from the plateau phase to resolution (body returning to its normal state) due to external circumstances such as an urgent phone call, a family member returning home or realizing you have run out of time and need to stop having sex. Parents may also recognize this scene from situations of being interrupted during love making by a toddler who has had a nightmare. In this case, your mind and body switches to focus on your child and you may or may not re-enter the desire and excitement phase when you return to bed. Or it may not be until the following day or later that the arousal process is reignited and continued. In addition, after orgasm, some people cycle back to further stimulation and experience further orgasms which is not addressed in this model.

As I have already mentioned, sometimes there are situations that might also hinder the arousal process from occurring as easily as this model suggests. Menopausal women may require more time for their body to produce enough lubrication. Some medications, for example, some types of antidepressants and even some hormonal birth control methods can hinder the body's response either through affecting hormone levels, libido, mood, lubrication or the ability to orgasm. Furthermore, if someone is stressed out and thinking about what their body looks like or all the work they need to do the following day, it is highly possible that they will also skip the orgasm phase.

However, being aware of the arousal phases can be a useful element in your understanding of your body and, at the same time, it can be just as useful to let go of the theory and focus on enjoying the sensations.

The elastic vagina

Is there such thing as too big? Because of my own vaginismus experience, I used to shake my head whenever I read about men being concerned about their penis not being big enough. In my opinion, big had been too big and smaller had always been better (and quite simply made sex possible). But eventually I learned that, except in very rare situations, a penis can't be 'too big' for a vagina.

The reality is that a vagina is very stretchy and can mold to fit around pretty much any penis size and open so wide as to allow a fully grown baby to pass through it. However, pain can occur during intercourse if the penis hits the entrance to the cervix or knocks an ovary, but this can be avoided or stopped by trying a position which doesn't result in deep thrusts or by the male choosing not to push in as deep. If a female feels she is too small, or the penis feels too wide, this is often a result of not being sufficiently aroused and lubricated and more time and care is required!

Talking about sex and pain, I'd also like to mention hymens and losing your virginity. The hymen is skin tissue at the entry to the vagina. It never completely covers the entrance even at birth and as a female ages through childhood into adolescence, it becomes thinner and the hole naturally widens as a result of everyday life. Many girls (as did I) however still fear the dreaded 'ripping' of their hymen when they lose their virginity and have been told that their first time will be painful because of this. Through proper sex education (if not in schools, then hopefully through knowledgeable adults, friends or resources online or elsewhere), young women should learn well before the time they become sexually active that the hymen is not thick enough to make sex impossible or even painful, but unfortunately even today many girls do not get adequate education on this topic.

There is obviously a wide range of reasons why the hymen = pain fallacy has circulated from one generation to the next in many societies spanning from religious teachings and beliefs to plain ignorance. Interestingly, it has been proved that this supposed ripping or breaking of the hymen generally doesn't even happen. It is also now established that having sexual intercourse shouldn't be a painful experience – yes ladies, not even the first time. Uncomfortable? Maybe. Not completely pleasurable? Sure. But, painful? No. (Unless of course you desire pain during sex, which some people find arousing in itself, but that's a whole different book!).

Pain upon first intercourse turns out to be a case of a self-fulfilling prophesy as anxiety and fear of expected pain heighten any discomfort, result in tense muscles and create pain. It is also a sad truth that many women do not choose their first time, but have it forced upon them – obviously not a relaxing experience at all! There was a reason why traditionally honeymoons lasted literally the time of a moon's cycle. It allowed the couple plenty of time to feel at ease and emotionally safe with one another and to explore and share their bodies in a sexual way. In an ideal world, a woman's first time would be with someone she trusts and feels comfortable and connected with emotionally as well as physically and there would be plenty of time for foreplay and pleasuring so that the woman is ready on all levels. If you have been having pain each time you have tried to have sex then slow down and don't rush things. Take your time and check whether you feel emotionally ready to take this step.

A note on orgasms

A good thing to know is that even if you have vaginismus, you can still have an orgasm. For many of you this probably goes without saying, but for some of us who experience vaginismus in our youth when we have little sexual experience to refer to, the thought that they might somehow be connected can come up.

That said, you may have to work on your ability to relax and be calm during intimate moments as it is apparently physically impossible for the female body to reach orgasm at the same time as being anxious. From an evolutionary viewpoint this, of course, makes perfect sense. It's more important for you to be aware of dangers in your environment and thus by fighting or escaping manage to survive than to have an orgasm. There are numerous exercises in this book that will help you enhance your ability to relax.

Many women find that they can learn first to orgasm on their own before they can with a partner. For me, it wasn't until years later that I started even really caring about or wanting an orgasm. And even then learning to have one was a step-by-step process that in itself took a number of years. First I learned how to orgasm when I was alone. Then I learned how to orgasm while with a partner and then how to incorporate it into intercourse.

Self-exploration and pleasuring through masturbation is a good way to become familiar with your personal preferences in terms of touch and what increases your level of arousal. If you are interested in reading more about masturbation, orgasms and techniques, you can read my book *Female Masturbation: Simple Pleasures to Mind-Blowing Orgasms* also available to purchase.

5. TREATING VAGINISMUS - IMPORTANT STEPS BEFORE YOU BEGIN THE EXERCISES

Now that you have an understanding of what can cause vaginismus, how it can persist as an automatic reaction, female arousal and loads of reasons why treating it is important for you, we come to what many of you will consider to be the most important part of this book: What to do to treat vaginismus.

The first step: See your doctor

The first logical step if you have been experiencing vaginismus is to check out with a doctor (preferably a gynecologist or a doctor who specializes in working with women's issues) whether it is actually vaginismus that you have. In addition, find out whether there is anything you are taking in terms of medication or birth control that might be having an affect on your vagina's ability to produce lubrication or affecting your arousal – all of which can lead to experiences of painful sex.

You can also check with your doctor whether doing the pelvic floor exercises later in the book (with the emphasis on learning to relax the muscles) is suitable for you.

Medications may be part of the problem

Anti-depressants and anti-anxiety medications are just two well known types of medications to have a negative impact on the sex lives of those who take them by decreasing sexual desire. This is a considerable problem in itself and there are many more prescription drugs and over the counter medications that also have this affect.

For the purposes of this book however, I am going to point out some of the medications that specifically dry up the vagina or affect physical arousal.

Medications that specifically affect arousal:
Allergy medications – Benadryl, Zyrtec, Claritin, Clarinex, and Alegra have the side effect of inhibiting arousal.
The Pill and DepoProvera inhibit arousal.
Pain relief medications: Advil, Aleve, Motrin, aspirin and numerous prescription-only drugs can inhibit arousal

Medications that specifically affect lubrication by drying the vagina:
Hypertension medications – Thiazide diuretics, and Beta blockers: Lopressor.
Allergy medications – those mentioned above also have the side effect of drying the vagina
Pain relief medications – those mentioned above also have the side effect of drying the vagina.
(Information taken from *Down there: Sexual and Reproductive Health*)

These are just some that I have come across that have these specific side effects. There are numerous medications that also affect sexual interest as well – too many to mention here. A general rule of thumb is to have a detailed read of the printouts that come with any prescription drugs you are taking as well as read the side effects of over-the-counter medications. In addition, your pharmacist and doctor are sources for more information.

Talking to a medical specialist and allowing them to take whatever tests they may require will allow you to rule out other pain-causing conditions caused by infection or inflammation as well as find out if it is in anyway age-related, for example, a side effect of menopause.

If your doctor tells you vaginismus doesn't exist (unfortunately some women have been told this), then I suggest you do some research and find another doctor. It's also possible that you are given a different diagnosis for what you are experiencing such as:

Dyspareunia: As mentioned earlier, this is the general medical term which means painful intercourse and is used to describe all types of sexual pain. Vaginismus is just one of the many possible causes of dyspareunia.

Vaginitis: Painful sex due to infection which may be resulting from sexually transmitted diseases or a yeast infection.

Vestibulodynia/vulvar vestibulitis: Pain upon touch at the sensitive area around the opening of the vagina which can lead to vaginismus.

Vulvodynia: Pain from a burning sensation in the vulva area due to irritation or hypersensitivity of the nerve fibers.

Even if you are given a different diagnosis from vaginismus or if you are told there is no physical cause to explain what is happening, there are still many useful lessons and exercises that you can benefit from in this book. Some people don't like being told "it's all in your head", whereas I tend to celebrate if I am ever told that because it means I can also fix it "with my head", by uncovering and healing underlying emotions, beliefs and learning whatever mind skills are required to promote healing.

The second step: Beliefs and emotions. What supports do you have?

The second step has to do with recognizing the sheer volume of possible limiting beliefs and emotions you may have built up over the years about sex, your vagina, sexuality, masturbation, what it means to be a female, etc. Just as I recommend going to a medical specialist to address any physical causes, I recommend finding an experienced therapist who can help you work through the emotional aspect of vaginismus and act as a supportive guide even as you take yourself through the self-help steps in this book. This is optional, but you might make faster, more effective and long-lasting change if you have support.

Busting beliefs – You can heal this!

Female arousal, sexuality, orgasms and masturbation

Regardless of how you were raised and the social background and time in history during which you have grown up, the reality is that orgasms and arousal are completely natural. So natural in fact that even babies do it! In her book *Sex Life: How our sexual experiences define who we are*, Dr Stephenson-Connolly describes how ultrasounds pick up erections in baby boys. Very young baby boys get erections and baby girls experience genital swelling and vaginal lubrication. And babies of both sexes have been observed masturbating to the point of orgasm even as young as four months old.

Obviously there is very little motor coordination at that age, however, a baby can rub against something, rock, tense its muscles and as Stephenson-Connolly highlights, these movements can lead to a "sudden release involving convulsions and rhythmic contractions – followed by noticeable relief and relaxation." It is important to note that babies engaging in such activity are not experiencing something in anyway similar to adult sexuality. A more appropriate way to think of such behavior is curious body exploration and enjoyment.

The unfortunate reality is that most parents do not know how to respond to a child's exploration or enjoyment and many people can remember a time of great confusion and shame upon being discovered touching 'their privates'. Over time, there can be a general acceptance that boys will be boys and that they will continue this self-exploration, but it is not generally accepted in females.

As a result, masturbation and talk of genitals is often more taboo for women than it is for men and this can be one of the attributing factors in vaginismus to explore for yourself. As you can see, these attitudes and feelings of awkwardness are learned; we are born with a natural curiosity and delight in our genitals and the joy they bring us.

Are you beginning to notice a raft of negative beliefs lurking within you? Thinking over the questions within this book will allow you to explore and challenge some of your own personal beliefs that are getting in the way of you having a fantastic sex life – the one you want. You might like to consider talking to a trusted friend or therapist about your answers as well.

Workbook questions:
What is your first memory of touching yourself?
Were you ever discovered touching your genitals as a child? What was the other person's reaction?
What were you taught about masturbation? What messages were you given (eg. it's fun, allowed, natural, something to do in private, shameful, disgusting, wrong?)
If you used to masturbate and you stopped, can you remember why?

Traumas can heal

Over the years, working as a therapist, I have worked with countless people supporting them in changing their emotional ties with old traumatic events. Again and again I am in awe at how quickly the intense emotional connection with a memory can be released even after the person has struggled with it for years.

At the same time it also makes sense that a person can experience a quick change in the way they feel. The brain and unconscious mind created the response very quickly back when someone first experienced a trauma and the mind is only holding onto the memory in that way because it is trying to keep you safe. The reality, however, is that this strategy is often flawed, leading people to live limited lives and avoid situations which in any way remind them of the original traumatic experience.

Once we address this unconscious need to keep safe, create a plan for moving forward and teach the mind a new way of storing that memory, there can be quite a rapid shift in the way that you remember it – in a way that is distant and removed, yet remembering everything that was positive and useful about the situation.

The most effective technique I have come across as a therapist for quickly and effectively healing trauma's comes from the field of NLP (Neuro Linguistic Programming). I have successfully used this process to help people overcome traumas ranging from rape and near-death-experiences during natural disasters, to relationship breakups, accidents and negative experiences in their childhood.

For some women, vaginismus starts after a traumatic experience such as sexual abuse. For others this is not the case; however, they may have traumatic memories of the times when they have attempted sex and experienced pain instead. For both situations, this NLP trauma healing process would be useful. See the section later in this book 'How to choose your health professionals'.

Beliefs can change

The great thing is that just as traumas can heal, beliefs can change. If you have beliefs about sex or about your body or yourself from your childhood or from your experiences with vaginismus, the comforting reality is that our beliefs can (and do) change over time. Beliefs that limit us in some way were – often unconsciously – created in the past and once we have become aware of them, how they limit us and what we would like to believe instead, we can begin to work on changing them.

Remember beliefs are not reality. They are just beliefs. That means we can change them!

Sometimes beliefs change when we get 'new' information or a new insight. I remember not being allowed to go to a party when I was a teenager – my mother banned me after I returned home late in the day after spending it with friends and not telling her when I would be back. I remember really hating her at that point; thinking she was so mean, so unreasonable and cruel. Much later in my twenties I remember talking to someone about her experience as a mother and how much she worried about her children and their well-being. In a flash, I recalled my earlier experience and noticed how my mind reformatted the meaning of my mother's actions. Suddenly, I saw the situation through her eyes. I imagined her worrying about my whereabouts and her concern and instantly my belief that she had acted unfairly changed. She still hadn't acted in a way that I was happy with at the time, but in my mind (due to my new found understanding and empathy), she wasn't a cruel person, but a stressed-out mother.

Again, there are many different therapeutic approaches out there for changing beliefs. One of the things you can do to facilitate this natural process is to provide yourself with factual information (about vaginismus for example) and a solid understanding of your situation. Reading this book will help with that. So too will the exploration of your beliefs and experiences in themselves. Keep exploring your sexuality by using the questions in this book as well as jotting down anything else that is sparked within you from the information. Remember you can address any beliefs that are holding you back with a therapist.

A big component is that it's a learned behavior

I have already talked about this and in greater detail in the earlier section 'Understanding vaginismus', but the beautiful reality about vaginismus is that no matter what the cause, a huge part of it (at least in it's continuation) comes down to it being a learned behavior. And just as nail-biters can stop biting their nails and people who hold tension in their jaw or shoulders can learn to relax those muscles and release tension and stress instead of storing it, you too can learn to relax your body and mind in order to have and enjoy sexual intercourse.

This is a really important factor in your healing journey: seeing vaginismus as something you can heal, as a response that you can retrain. Vaginismus is a highly treatable condition with a high rate of success when people fully commit to working on both the psychological and physical aspects of it. So all you have to do is decide to be one of those people and then follow the steps that the experts recommend.

Okay, so hopefully you've taken the first two steps – first, checked your physical health with a doctor and second, at least considered getting support from someone you trust for the underlying emotions, if not found a therapist and booked your first session. For help on choosing health professionals, I have included some tips later in the book on what you should look for.

6. PART TWO: EXERCISES: REDUCING TENSION IN YOUR BODY - BREATHWORK, BODY AWARENESS AND WORKING WITH A PARTNER

Reducing tension in your body is one of the most important components in stopping the vaginismus response. Therefore, I have selected the best relaxation-promoting exercises for you and put them in a logical order. These exercises will help you progress through touch and body awareness experiences so that your body and mind learn how to relax and enjoy touch. These are exercises that I have found useful myself (even after the vaginismus was 'gone' I still had numerous issues I had to work through). Exercises such as these helped me in becoming completely at ease with my body and during intimacy through to sexual intercourse. Other exercises, such as the ones using vaginal dilators, I did not personally have to use, however they are well documented as useful for those who do decide to use them.

Body work: How to reduce tension in your body.

Vaginismus at a purely physical level is all about tension as a result of your body's response and as a flow-on effect of your thoughts. So all of these exercises will teach you how to release this tension and become more relaxed. Breathing is one way of effectively releasing tension and once you get good at doing that, you should be able to stop the tension in its tracks. These breathing techniques you can then use while being physically intimate with a partner. But that comes later!

1. Breathwork: Belly breathing

Watch a baby or an animal sleeping and notice where breathing takes place in their body. Observing them in their stillness you will see that they breathe all the way down to their belly. There is little to no raising of the shoulders, and the stomach area literally moves in and out as the lungs fill with air and empty on every breath.

Many people unlearn this natural way of breathing (called 'diaphragmatic breathing') whether through being told to "stand up, shoulders back, stomach in", through attempts to look slim by sucking in their stomach, through hours of ballet training or as an anxiety response which in itself promotes shallow breathing. If you are fortunate to have had singing lessons or learned to play a wind instrument then you will have learned the proper use of your diaphragm and how to breathe deeply. Don't worry, to get the most out of the exercises in this book you don't need to know anything about your diaphragm. For those of you who are curious, it is a muscle that extends across the bottom of your rib cage. When you breathe in deeply (i.e. properly) the diaphragm descends, pressing down on the stomach and causing it to bulge out. As you breathe out, the diaphragm relaxes and rises and your stomach flattens again.

Belly breathing: 6-10 minutes

1. Lie down on your back.

2. Place one or both hands on your stomach near your belly button.

3. Breathe normally and notice how deep you are breathing and whether your belly is rising with each intake.

4. Take some time to consciously choose to slow down your breathing and breathe more deeply until you feel the rise and fall of your stomach.

5. Stay in this position and continue this way of breathing for a minimum of 5 minutes, or longer if you wish.

6. Afterward, take note how you are feeling compared to when you first lay down. If you have lowered your breathing from the upper chest area down to your belly, then you should be feeling more relaxed. Well done!

Full lung breathing: 6-10 minutes

1. Stand or sit with a straight back.

2. Place one hand on your belly button and another on your chest.

3. Breathe and notice which hands are rising and falling naturally. Just notice.

4. Now start to slow down your breathing and breathe more deeply.

5. Focus on creating a movement in both hands. More so in your belly, but also some rise in your chest as your lungs fill. The key movement you are aiming for is still in your stomach.

6. Stay in this position and continue this way of breathing for a minimum of 5 minutes, longer if you wish.

7. Take note afterward how you are feeling compared to when you first started.

Angel wings breathing: 1– 2 minutes

If you are flexible enough you can test this yourself, however, you may require someone else's help. This exercise is another way to check the depth of your breathing. If you are breathing properly, you will be able to feel the movement of the diaphragm in your lower back and flanks (the sides of your waist between hip and ribs).

1. Rest an arm along your lower back or get someone to place their hands there.

2. Place your other hand on one of your sides at waist height.

3. Breathe as with the earlier exercises and attempt to create a noticeable movement in these areas.

The 4,7,8 breathing pattern

There are many different breathing techniques you can learn to reduce the stress and anxiety response. Often the roots of these breathing techniques are in spiritual teachings such as Zen Buddhism, Yoga, and Taoism. In the modern day world, psychologists are increasingly reaching for this ancient wisdom and teaching these techniques to their clients as they are a simple take-home tool. Some are easier to learn than others. One that has proven especially effective for myself over the years as well as for clients who have used it as a simple tool to help them get to sleep and to calm themselves down in the middle of a panic attack is the 4,7,8 breathing pattern.

Practice this daily once you are sure that you have established belly breathing as your normal way of breathing. As the increase in oxygen intake can lead to a little lightheadedness when you are new to this, I suggest you only do four rounds of the 4,7,8 technique when you start off. You can slow down the speed of your counting after you have become familiar with the pattern and a nice way of tying it in with mindfulness and body awareness is to use your heartbeat to decide the speed of the counts.

First learn and practice this breathing method when you don't need it, i.e., when you are already relaxed. Then you will be able to draw on it in the future to focus on and do when feeling anxious and tense.

1. Breathe in through your nose for the count of four.

2. Hold the breath for the count of seven.

3. Breathe out for the count of eight through your mouth

making an "ahhhh" or "whoosh" sound.

4. Immediately breathe in through the nose again for the count of four and repeat the hold for seven and breathe out for eight.

You might be asking yourself: 'How long is a count?' Well, the simple answer to that is that a count is as long or as short as you want it to be. It's as simple as that! Just make sure you are keeping a regular count. When you first try this exercise, you may like to use a faster count and as you get better at it, you can slow the counts down as you get better at using your full lung capacity.

Tip: A particularly peaceful way I have found to do this exercise is to use my heart beat as the count.

2. Body awareness

With all of the following exercises, it is of top most importance that you feel in control of your experience. That means you need to set aside time when you know that you will not be disturbed. You should also ensure you have a private, secure space where you can relax.

That means turning off phones and other devices that might otherwise distract you, asking to not be interrupted if you live with others, locking any doors, and making sure you have time set aside. I don't recommend attempting these exercises in the middle of a busy day or knowing you need to rush off straight afterward.

To get the best possible results, do what you can to make the space feel comfortable. You might like to create a beautiful atmosphere. This is a date with yourself, so go ahead and set the scene. Light candles, heat essential oils or burn incense, warm the room if required. All of this is optional and a personal choice. Candles and the like don't appeal to everyone so do what feels right to you.

These exercises can be done at any time and in any body position, but for starters I want you to take some time out and do them lying down. It is also useful to do them lying down for the sheer obviousness that often sex and other sexually related exercises that come later in this book will be undertaken in a lying position. Plus lying down in itself is a relaxing position and I want you to feel relaxed while doing these exercises.

Mindfulness

Mindfulness is a term used to describe the act of just noticing in a relaxed way what is going on around you and within you without judgment or any attempt to guide your thoughts in a certain direction.

Mindfulness these days is often spoken of with reference to its Buddhist roots, but it also has a history in Christianity (I've heard it referred to as simply 'having awareness'). In fact, many of the spiritual practices around the world that I have read about include some form of mindfulness (going by a different name perhaps) in their teachings. It can bring a great sense of mental and spiritual calm to those who regularly practice. Neuroscience and medical research have also shown that entering a space of calm awareness plays a significant role in healing emotional and physical traumas as well as enhancing health.

This is an exercise which is all about awareness without judgment. Tuning into your current experience and choosing what you focus on – where your attention is, is a vital skill for developing a positive sexual experience and sex life. I can't emphasize that enough. So many people with issues and negative emotions associated with sex find themselves anywhere but in the moment while having sex – even if it is with a trusted long-term partner. They find their minds wandering into the past, recalling negative experiences and replaying them or looking into the immediate future and creating scenes in which they are anxious and feeling pain. In some instances, people mentally leave their body completely. This is a typical response during a traumatic experience such as sexual abuse – by tuning out, the subconscious protects you from having to consciously experience the abuse. Unfortunately, this tuning out (in psychology speak called dissociation), often continues in subsequent safe, consensual sexual situations – much to the frustration of the person reacting in this way.

So here are the steps:

1. Lie down and get comfortable.

2. Tell yourself that you are going to take some time to 'just be'.

3. Take some time noticing your current experience through each of your senses.

4. What sounds can you hear?

5. What sensations do you feel – inside your body, against you body, textures, temperatures?

6. What can you see just by moving your eyes while

keeping your head still and relaxed?

7. What can you smell? Even if you haven't added any smells through the burning of incense or essential oils, you can still notice what smells might be present. From lingering smells from a meal to the smell of a partner in the bed sheets, to a flower's scent wafting through an open window.

8. And tastes? What can you taste in your mouth? Anything noticeable?

9. And back to other senses again, feeling your breath – however which way you are breathing.

10. Notice that thoughts also drift through your mind as you lie here. You might be feeling silly or uncomfortable or calm and restful. You might be thinking about work or your shopping list or noticing the ceiling needs repainting.

11. Allow these thoughts to drift in and out of your mind as you observe them coming and going. All of this is fine and doesn't matter.

12. None of it matters right now.

13. Just bring your attention back to the here and now and the many things you are experiencing through your senses.

14. Take a little time to adjust yourself back to the room properly and get up when you wish.

Body scanning

This can be done at any time and in any body position, but at least for the first time you do this, I want you to focus fully on the exercise and follow the steps while lying down.

1. Lie down on your back.

2. Take a few minutes to become aware of your breath and adjust to belly breathing if you haven't already.

3. Become attuned to the here and now and your sensory experiences as you did in the mindfulness exercise.

4. Starting at your toes, and moving up your body all the way through to the top of your head and tips of your fingers, scan through the various areas and notice where you feel heavy and relaxed and which areas hold tension.

5. While breathing deeply, pause at areas that hold tension, imagining you are breathing in to release the tension there. Allow the muscles to relax and sink further into the surface you are lying on. Relax and let go.

6. Continue scanning, pausing and relaxing whereever there is a need in your body.

7. Repeat throughout your entire body two or more times allowing yourself and choosing to let go of any remaining tension.

8. The more often you repeat this exercise over time, the better you will get at noticing tension, choosing to release it and relax deeper with your breath.

Progressive muscle relaxation

As I mentioned earlier, from a physical perspective vaginismus is all about holding tension – more specifically about unconsciously holding or creating tension. And just as people who unconsciously tense their jaw or shoulders can learn to regain awareness and control over being able to actively relax these areas, you can gain control over your vaginal muscles through specific muscle relaxation exercises. Learning to relax your *whole* body is also very important, because you need to learn to feel relaxation throughout your whole body when having sexual intercourse without the vaginismus reaction.

1. Lie down on your back.

2. Start at your feet and toes. Flex and tense your toes and feet.

3. Hold the tension for a few seconds and then let go of it and relax. Allow yourself to take a deep breath in and out.

4. Move your focus to your legs. Tense your feet first and now tense the muscles in your legs as well.

5. Let go and breathe.

6. Tense your feet, your legs, your butt muscles and pelvic area including the muscles you use to stop the flow of urine.

7. Let go and breathe.

8. Tense your feet, legs, butt and pelvis and now also your stomach and back.

9. Let go and breathe.

10. Tense the muscles again, this time adding in your shoulders.

11. Let go and breathe.

12. Now add neck and face – really scrunch up your face.

13. Let go and breathe.

14. Now add arms and hands. Clench your fists and arms.

15. Let go and breathe.

16. Repeat all muscles and then relax and breathe.

17. Take a few deep breaths. Notice how much more calm you feel and how much heavier and relaxed your body is now. Well done!

Finding your erogenous zones

Women who experience vaginismus in part due to not being fully aroused can do themselves a huge favor by identifying their personal erogenous zones or "sensitive spots" as I like to call them. This will give you an understanding of what kind of touch you enjoy where and knowing that, you can also tell or teach your partner.

I can't stress this often enough to my clients: Your partner is not a mind reader! Do not expect that they will automatically know what turns you on. Even if you have been together for years, if you have never told them they will still have many things they can learn about you.

Once you have a good understanding of these areas on your body which feel ultra nice to be touched, then you can communicate and ask your partner to touch you there, and in the way you like, when you are being intimate together.

I don't want you to try to make this experience with yourself sexual, just sensual. Ideally, you will do this undressed in a warm room, but you can also experiment while wearing a light layer of clothes.

Really take your time to gently draw lines along all the areas on your body that you can reach. You will need to move about for this exercise to be able to reach some of the areas. Just focus on areas that are easily reachable – this is not a time to break out any stretches!

Enjoy and play around any sensitive areas that you find. Draw circles and lines and notice how different pressures increase or decrease the enjoyment and feelgood quality of the touch. Close your eyes and breathe deeply. Come from a space of love and awe at the magnificence of the human body, your body – and the pleasure it can give you.

Even though we are all unique, but there are certain areas which are erogenous zones for many women, so here are some ideas for you to start out with from top to bottom:

Ears
Lips
Nipples and breasts
Neck – front and back
Lower back
Inner arm
Palm of hand

Vulva – lips and clitoris
Inner thigh
Ankle
Soles of feet

Afterward, you might like to take some time to jot down some of the areas you discovered are your favorite erogenous zones. Perhaps you even discovered one or two that surprised you. When I did this, I was fascinated to discover that often my most pleasantly sensitive spots were also those where I am the most ticklish. I guess that makes sense, but it was quite an eye-opener for me at the time – it's not that I don't want to be touched there, just softly!

Another interesting discovery for me was that just by becoming more aware of my erogenous zones, they became more sensitive over time leading to increased pleasure.

Workbook questions:
What areas were you surprised to discover are included in your erogenous zones?
What are your most sensitive spots and areas you got the most pleasure from?

PC muscle training

Some studies using electromyography (EMG), a technique which measures the electrical activity of muscles during contraction and at rest, have shown vaginismus sufferers to have pelvic floor muscles that even in their resting state are partially contracted (clenched). Furthermore these muscles have shown to clench in vaginismus sufferers more easily, much in the way that others may unconsciously frown or tense their jaw when stressed.

These findings differ slightly from theories that emphasize the anxiety response cycle whereas the EMG findings indicate that the cause is a simple muscle overcompensation. Now those of you who in the past have been able to have sexual intercourse with someone and now cannot or who can easily insert a tampon or fingers but not a penis will know that it is not a simple case of muscles overworking and that there is more to it for you. This theory might make sense for some of my readers though.

However, the following steps for healing vaginismus are the same regardless. Gaining control over muscle contraction and relaxation is the key.

The following pelvic floor muscle training exercise, often called Kegel or PC exercises, are the same recommended for women who need to gain or regain bladder control, for example after childbirth. These exercises are also practiced worldwide by women wanting to increase their orgasmic response and create a tighter grip on their partner's penis during intercourse which increases feelings of pleasure in both partners.

Of course for women experiencing vaginismus, the focus and important aspect of the exercise is to gain control over these vaginal muscles as well as learn how to consciously relax and release any tension. These exercises are one part of the journey of learning to have conscious control so that you are eventually able to relax them during sexual intercourse or penetration.

1. To prepare for the following exercise, first locate your

PC muscle by stopping your urine flow while peeing.

2. Once you know which muscle to squeeze, you can practice exercising your PC muscle anywhere. Don't worry if you are exercising not just your PC muscle but including more of the pelvic floor/vaginal muscles. The main thing is that you will be learning to relax the muscles in your vaginal area.

3. For starters, while sitting, lying or standing, take a deep breath in and then squeeze this muscle and hold for the count of three.

3. Breathe out and relax the muscle (in the same way you learned in the progressive muscle relaxation exercise).

4. Repeat daily in repetitions of 15 quick squeeze and release combinations with the focus on the release and relaxation of the muscle.

5. Practice twice a day. You can increase the number of squeeze-and-release sets you do, but the main purpose for you is to regain control over the muscle. For one set continue the quick hold and release pattern and for the second session squeeze and hold for a longer count e.g. five seconds, and then on the exhale release and relax your body fully.

6. Continuing these exercises at a fixed time is the easiest way to remember to do them e.g. while brushing your teeth or before you go to sleep or even while driving to work. The best thing about PC exercises is that no-one can tell you are doing them and you can do them anytime and anywhere.

Dilator therapy

Not everyone will want or even need to take this step, however the use of vaginal dilators offers a practical approach and is often part of comprehensive treatment programs. If you do decide to purchase dilators make sure that you are buying medical-grade dilators from a reputable source. Again, this is something I recommend you discuss with your health professional. He or she will be able to give a professional opinion on whether dilator therapy would be useful for you as well as direct you to a trusted manufacturer.

Vaginal dilators are therapeutic devices that come in various sizes (often sold in sets) for insertion into the vagina, allowing the user to practice controlling and activating a relaxed pelvic floor while penetrated, working up from thinner to wider sizes. Dilators look similar to basic vibrators, and they come in a range of sizes.

How to use and incorporate them into your healing process: Allow for at least 30 minutes each time you do dilator exercises as this allows not only for the 15-minute period of holding the dilator inside your vagina, but also some time beforehand to get into a calm state of mind and relax your body.

1. As with most of these experiences, ensuring you have time and privacy is of utmost importance.

2. Lie down on your back.

3. Using your skills learned from the earlier muscle relaxation exercises, scan your body and breathe deeply into any areas where your muscles are tense. You may

find using the progressive muscle relaxation method of first clenching and then releasing the tension in each area of muscles easier. Focus especially on the pelvic area, relaxing your buttocks, thighs and stomach muscles.

4. Taking the smallest dilator, apply some lubricant (this could be bought lubricant or you could use your saliva) to the tip of the dilator and vaginal entrance.

5. Place the dilator against the vaginal entrance.

6. While maintaining deep breathing, slide the dilator in as far as is comfortable. This might be only a few centimeters or it might be half or even completely in.

7. Pause and do not push it in any further if you feel any pain or discomfort.

8. As well as focusing on physically relaxing your muscles and keeping calm through the diaphragmatic breathing, you can increase comfort through the use of your imagination. Visualize your vaginal walls as stretchy and loose and relaxed. Remind yourself that you are in control and that you are choosing to relax and allow your vagina to accommodate the dilator inside you.

9. With every exhale, relax and release your muscles further and, at your own pace and comfort, insert the dilator further if it is not already, until it is fully inserted.

10. Keep your body relaxed and your breathing deep.

11. Leave the dilator inside you for 15 minutes at a time while you rest and relax.

12. Once 15 minutes have passed, gently remove the dilator and wash it according to the manufacturer's

instructions.

13. You may benefit from taking some extra time after removing the dilator to reflect on your experience. Some women may wish to keep a journal to record their experiences and progress. You could also talk about it with a loved one or trusted therapist.

If you are going to go to the effort of purchasing and using dilators, then it makes sense to get the most out of them. This means committing to daily practice of holding one inside your vagina for 15 minutes. In your own time you will progress through the sizes to the wider dilators as you get full control over relaxing your pelvic floor muscles and feel fully comfortable with each size. Once you have reached the stage of comfortable insertion and holding of the size you choose (or for heterosexual women, the size of your partner's penis), you may be ready for intercourse. Make sure to practice the sensate focusing exercises with your partner before recommencing sexual intercourse.

Variations

You can also progress from simply holding the dilator inside your vagina including movements such as rotations, insertion and withdrawal, from side to side and increasing how far you have inserted it. However, start by doing the basic routine of simply inserting it and staying in a relaxed state.

Alternative to dilators: You may find that time alone exploring with a slim vibrator, in a similar fashion to the dilator exercise above, can be enough as you learn to relax during penetration. The difference the use of a vibrator makes is that you can take advantage of it's vibrating function, if you wish, to help you become aroused and naturally lubricated. It's up to you. For some women, it is preferable to practice in a non-sexual way, while others might like the variation. Again, do what feels best for you.

Masturbation

Masturbation is a great healing and learning tool for many women as well as a useful way to release sexual tension, and access physical relaxation and pleasure. In the case of treating vaginismus, it can be an extremely helpful factor in the overcoming of emotional and psychological causes behind the condition.

Self-pleasuring puts the sexual experience 100% in your hands and you thus have full control. For anyone anxious about sexual intercourse and the interaction with a sexual partner, this alone time with your sexual side is extremely useful for being able to explore and discover without fear of external pressure or judgment. Self-pleasuring helps you become at ease with your body and your arousal and what works for you.

There are many ways you can pleasure yourself from rubbing yourself against a pillow, to caressing your clitoris and vaginal lips (labia) with your fingers to the incorporation of sex toys such as a simple vibrator. There is no right way to masturbate and each individual has their own personal preferences that they discover, just as we each have preferences about making love, where and how we like to be touched, etc.

Just as having an active sex life is your choice, so too is whether you choose to masturbate or not. It's up to you.

Many women grow up with the message that touching themselves 'down there' is somehow wrong or dirty and they carry those messages with them through their whole lives. Some women got taught those messages in a way that was not obvious and they remain largely unconscious, with the individual just noticing that it feels 'not right' in some way. Some women are embarrassed about masturbation. If you are embarrassed, then you may wish to confront and release negative thoughts or beliefs that have been passed on to you during your childhood, thus enabling yourself to freely explore the joys of masturbation. Or you might want to release them so that you are free as an individual to choose for yourself (without old chains restricting you in any way).

You may be interested in my book *Female Masturbation: Simple Pleasures to Mind-Blowing Orgasms* if you want more details about masturbation and orgasms. Reading more about this topic may also help you realize you can let go of old teachings still hanging around from your childhood.

Workbook questions:
How do you find the experience of pleasuring yourself?
If it was your first time how was it just now?
What is easy about it for you?
What do you enjoy about it?
Is there anything that feels like a challenge – physically or emotionally?
What have you learned about yourself
What might you look forward to next time?
What could be enjoyable to try out next time?

3. Working with a partner

On an emotional level, vaginismus is about anxiety – the arch-enemy of relaxation. However, relaxation is crucial to being able to enjoy a full sexual experience with another person. If you are in a long term relationship and have vaginismus, you and your partner could benefit from him/her also attending sessions with any therapists and/or specialists you consult as your partner will be having to work with you in order to make progress. Having your partner's understanding and support will make a huge difference in how easy or challenging the process will be.

The stronger and more closely connected you feel as a couple, the more comfortable and safe you will feel to be able to work through exercises as well as build on a strong foundation of gentle intimacy for when you progress to intercourse.

Notice I said *progress to intercourse*. If you are currently having painful penetrative sex then I recommend you stop as of today and for the time being focus on these exercises until you are ready to attempt intercourse again. Remember, the tricky thing with vaginismus is that even if you love your partner and even if you feel comfortable with them already, if your vagina clenches during attempts of penetration then you perpetuate the cycle by continuing this biofeedback loop. You need to learn to gain full control over your relaxation – alone and with a partner.

Eye gazing: 2-5 minutes

Looking deep into each others eyes has a number of interesting effects. People often say that it reconnects them with feelings of love for their partner. That's not surprising as studies have shown strangers to feel more emotionally connected to people with whom they have had to do this exercise with for as little as a couple of minutes.

How to eye-gaze: As the name of the exercise suggests, simply get into a comfortable position and look into each others eyes for a while. I have suggested the duration of a couple to five minutes, but there's no real time limit for this.

Doing this exercise while holding hands could be a simple way to start any further exercises and experiences of intimacy while you are progressing along your journey.

If one of you feels uncomfortable at any time, simply close your eyes for a little bit and then re-engage.

You can do this exercise in any position so long as you are facing each other and are comfortable enough to be able to maintain eye contact.

Questions to answer after the exercise: How was that for each of you? What thoughts and emotions came up? How did it feel the second or third time you did it?

Repeat this exercise until you feel comfortable looking into each others eyes for at least two minutes. The experience of uninterrupted eye gazing is a technique you can then use if needing to pause during any challenging exercises or moments of intimacy to emotionally touch base and refocus together.

Breathing in time: 5-10 minutes each

Any couple can benefit from the experience of taking turns to be held and being nurtured. In particular, couples with intimacy difficulties will find it creates a deeper bond and safe attachment. Because the following exercise mimics the position of a caring parent and child, some people find this an extremely powerful and healing exercise, especially if they did not get consistent love and support during their childhood.

Breathing in time - as outlined in this exercise, or reciprocal breathing where one person breathes in as the other breathes out ('breathing the one breath') are just two out of numerous breathing techniques with their roots in Tantra. The following simplified version I came across in Stella Resnick's book *The Heart of Desire*, however there are more complex Tantra versions which go further into channeling the energy between you and your lover's body.

How to do this exercise:

1. Lie down in a position where one of you can rest their head against their partner's chest and the other can hold them in their arms. Support the neck and any other areas requiring propping up with pillows or cushions. I will refer to these two positions as the holder and the one being held.

2. The person being held has only one thing to do in this task and that is to relax into the other persons arms and feel their loving embrace.

3. The holder has the task of breathing in time with the person they are holding. The breath can be sensed through the rise and fall in areas such as their belly and chest. If you find it hard to feel the breathing rate of your partner when you are the holder, then you can simply ask your partner to make an audible sound as they breathe out. This doesn't have to be a big sighing sound or anything similar. An out breath can simply be made louder by slightly opening the mouth and letting the breath become audible as the air passes the lips.

4. Swap roles and once each of you has had a turn share your experiences of being the holder and the one being held.

Sharing your experience with your partner helps to creates a deeper bond and more understanding between you:

How was it to be held like that and having the other person breathe in time with you?
How was it to hold and focus on breathing in time with the other person?

Sensate focusing

You have already explored some sensate exercises for individual exploration earlier in the book as you explored your body and tuned into your physical sensations and experience of the moment. Developed by Masters and Johnson, the following sensate focusing exercises are an effective way to relearn safe sexual touch with a partner. As the name implies, the following exercises have the purpose of increasing awareness and pleasure of the sensual experience rather than viewing it as sexual. This doesn't mean that you will not get aroused during the exercises. But the focus is not on sex (and thus the pressure to perform or act in a certain way). There is also a chance that any fears and anxiety around sex you may have might be triggered by these exercises. Thus, it is recommended that you give yourselves plenty of undisturbed time for the exercises as well as comforting and discussion afterward. You may also choose to work through any issues that arise with a therapist.

Remember while doing sensate focusing that the purpose is to enhance your sexual relationship through the positive and caring experience of becoming more in tune with each other's bodies and responses to touch. Touching while naked yet 'starting afresh' as if getting to know each other for the first time also helps rewire the brain and unconscious to feel comfortable during sexual intercourse.

Each stage is separate and takes place over a period of time. The recommended pace of progression through the stages is dictated by the comfort of the couple. More specifically, wait until you are both at ease at the current stage and feel emotionally ready to continue to the next, more intimate, stage. Ideally, you will set aside time regularly each week to give and receive touch via the sensate focusing exercises. This could be 1 hour per week (30 minutes each). Or more frequently but for shorter times such as three times weekly for 10 minutes each giving and receiving.

Stage 1:

At stage one, you take turns to touch each other's body – anywhere except for the breasts and genital areas. Agree on a specific amount of time for each of you to have a turn as the 'toucher' such as 10 minutes. Apart from letting each other know if any touch is uncomfortable, the task is to be as quiet as possible and to simply be mindful and present of the experience of touching or being touched without any sexual agenda. If arousal happens, do NOT engage in sexual intercourse. The focus is to stay with this non-sexual, sensual touch. At this stage, kissing is also out of bounds.

Stage 2:

Again taking turns, this time areas that can be touched include breasts and genitals. Kissing is also allowed from this stage on. However, these areas are not to become the primary focus of the touch nor should there be an attempt to arouse the your partner. The task is to keep the purpose of the touch on awareness of physical sensations. Intercourse and orgasm are both still out of bounds at this stage, even if one or both of you want it.

Another addition at this stage is clear non-verbal communication through the person being touched placing their hand on top of the touching hand and expressing when they would like more or less pressure, speed or a change in body area. The flow and touch however, is still being initiated by the 'toucher'. They still follow their interests in touching rather than the person being touched taking over.

Stage 3:

Only after competing the first two stages successfully (remaining calm, relaxed and enjoying being touched and touching your partner) should you progress to stage three. In this stage, you allow yourselves to touch in a way that is more natural – touch each other simultaneously rather than with any clear boundaries of whose turn it is.

Again, regardless of how sexually aroused either of you may feel as a result of this exercise, sexual intercourse is still NOT allowed.

Stage 4:

At this stage, you continue practicing touching each other simultaneously. The progression at this stage is that once you feel comfortable, you can move into a position where you are on top of your partner. You can experiment with moving between sitting and lying positions as well as explore rubbing your vulva, clitoris and vaginal opening against your partner's genitals. If your partner is a male, you can explore this genital to genital contact and rubbing whether he has an erection or not.

Stage 5:

Starting with simultaneous touching and progressing to the woman on top position, you decide the amount of genital on genital contact. When you feel comfortable and your partner has an erection you can guide the penis to the entrance of your vagina. If your partner is a female, you could guide one or more of her fingers inside you.

If there are, at any point, feelings of discomfort or anxiety, simply acknowledge them to yourself as well as let your partner know and move back to non-genital touching.

Stage 6:

After a couple of times at step 5, many couples feel comfortable enough to continue on to intercourse. Again, it is important that you decide when you feel ready for this next step. Remember, at any of these stages you can take a step back to an earlier stage if you feel the need to.

Questions to answer and discuss together after the sensate focusing exercises:
How do you find each stage?
What is easy about each stage?
What is a challenge?
What have you learned about yourself?
What have you learned about your partner?
What are you looking forward to next time?

Dilator use with your partner

If you choose to include dilators in your healing program, you can decide to include your partner in the exercises with the dilator.

Some variations of this could be:

– Including them right from the start – allowing them to provide emotional comfort and support at specific times along the stages of increasing the size.

– Having them join you once you have had a lot of practice and feel comfortable inserting and holding a wider dilator.

– Once you can easily insert, hold and move the dilator inside you, your partner could take the role of inserting and moving it under your instruction. This is an option, which I recommend once you have mastered the following abilities: Diaphragmatic breathing and consciously relaxing your muscles (including your pelvic floor muscles). It is also important that you feel confident that you will be able to direct the process with your partner. I also recommend that you have completed all other partner exercises in this book with your partner before you do this.

7. PART THREE: INCORPORATING YOUR LEARNINGS INTO SEX WITH A PARTNER

Sex therapists agree that persisting with painful penetration and sex which is painful in any way is not recommended and can lead to further physical and psychological difficulties. Always remember that you have the right to say "no" or "stop!" And if you continue to feel pain during sex even after doing the exercises in this book, I cannot stress enough how important it is to speak to a health professional! With a proper diagnosis you can rule out or treat any physical issues and have the peace of mind that comes from being able to understand your situation. If you are embarrassed, then reminding yourself that they are doctors and talk about this kind of stuff with patients all the time might be helpful.

By doing the partner exercises included in this book you

have already started to incorporate and merge the things you have learned with sexual intimacy.

Over time, in order to continue deepening your ease with your partner and your sexual intimacy, keep up the clear communication – during times of intimacy (unless requested to remain quiet such as in the early sensate focusing exercises) as well as other times during the day, letting your partner know how you feel and how far you think you have progressed in your healing journey.

Follow the exercises that suit your situation, speak to any health professionals you have chosen to work with and consider yourself and your own needs and desires as well as your partner's. Checking in with yourself like this means that you can map out your next steps – the ones that work at a pace that feels right for you. On a really positive note, of the many pain-during-sex related conditions, vaginismus is regarded as one that responds extremely well to treatment with most women being able to eventually have pain free intercourse.

Key points for creating sexual arousal

Your body has numerous erogenous zones, many of which you have hopefully by now discovered during your own solo exploration as well as during the sensate focusing exercises with your partner (that is if you currently have one). Bringing this knowledge into the bedroom and taking time to tune in with each other's bodies through gentle touch can help a woman relax, become aroused and feel comfortable to progress to more direct sexual touch.

In addition to non-genital erogenous zones, there are recognized trigger points or 'hot spots' on the woman's body that when stimulated are particularly effective in increasing a woman's arousal levels. If you want to gain more understanding of trigger points and their resulting orgasms, I explore this topic in full detail in my ebook *Female Masturbation: Simple Pleasures to Mind-Blowing Orgasms*. There are a number of key areas on the female body as well as other significant factors for creating sexual arousal that you should definitely be aware of, so I'll point a few of them out here as well.

Clitoris: A spot that most people are familiar with and associate with female arousal is the clitoris. This highly sensitive organ (which actually extends deep within the vagina) is a easy place to start. The clitoris is proof that sex is supposed to be an experience of enjoyment for a woman as its only role is that of being a source of pleasure!

You will have to let your partner know what feels pleasing for you in terms of the speed and pressure of touch on the clitoris as each woman is different. Don't expect your partner to be a mind-reader and somehow know what you would like them to do without telling them. For many, an ultra light touch on the bulb or ball-like protrusion at the top of the vaginal lips can be very arousing, as can increasing the pressure and/or speed according to your arousal or varying the touch or source of touch (e.g. your partner's fingers, tongue or lips).

U-spot: Another area that is very sensitive and increases a woman's arousal is the u-spot, which is the area running between the inner lips from the clitoral bulb to the vaginal opening. Gentle caresses with fingers or mouth can be very arousing. Again, let your partner know what you would like and what works for you.

G-spot: This much spoken about 'spot' is a sensitive area on the front vaginal wall (closest to the front of your body). People often learn to access this area in their partner by using a 'come hither' motion with their fingers. Stimulation of the g-spot can produce intense orgasms and female ejaculation. Hard to reach by yourself, this is a spot your partner can stimulate for you, or you could use a curved vibrator specifically designed to stimulate the g-spot. If you are still working on making penetration possible, then this is an experience you can save for later.

A woman's biggest sex organ: Her mind

On the one hand we have these body areas like the u-spot and clitoris as well as breasts and all the other places that feel exquisite when touched, but the reality is that female arousal is not just a physical matter. Much to the frustration of many a man, the female body is not like a computer or robot which reacts at the touch of a button. A female's arousal process is quite complex and whoever said that the mind is a woman's biggest sex organ sure knew what they were talking about.

Have you heard the joke about 'foreplay starts with the morning dishes'? Well actually it's true! Men who do their share (as perceived by the woman) of the housework often get more sex. Why? It has to do with a woman feeling valued and not taken advantage of. We like to be considered and our work appreciated. So too do men by the way!

But asking your partner to do more of the housework is

just one possible option and rather limiting – what happens if they don't do it or they can't? Again, I'm going to promote self-responsibility. Rather than putting full responsibility for your arousal on your partner, think for yourself about what gets you in the mood and helps you feel interested in sexual intimacy.

Some ideas to increase your arousal

– Women can be self-conscious about their bodies during intimate interactions. If this is you, support your comfort by purchasing some candles that will create soft lighting that is flattering or make good use of dimmers or fireplaces.

– Buy lingerie or sleepwear that fits and flatters your body shape and size. Go ahead and ask for assistance in the shop when buying lingerie if you are not sure – they are trained to know what will suit you!

– Set dates with your partner. This is counterintuitive; you might think that planning to have sex or to be intimate would decrease arousal because it is the opposite of spontaneity. However, planning actually increases arousal for many women as the anticipation can be a turn on in itself – especially when you know the focus during your 'date' will be on caring, loving touch. Planning to be intimate also means that you can do things that make you feel more in the mood like wearing something you feel attractive in and showering or brushing teeth or even eating foods for dinner that won't cause your belly to bloat.

– Look after your body; eat well, exercise, get regular time in the sun and nature to get enough vitamin D and relax, wear clothes that are comfortable and in colors you like and that suit you, get enough sleep and time out.

What if I'm single?

If you are single you may feel like you're at a disadvantage in your healing journey since you don't have a partner to work with on the partner exercises. While there are some exercises you may have to skip, the reality is that you have more than enough exercises to work on – from the breathing and relaxation exercises to the physical body exploration exercises and working through your emotions and negative beliefs.

Actually, the way I see it, you have the advantage of being able to focus purely on yourself and really give yourself the time and loving attention required without having to worry at all about your partner's needs while you work through these exercises. In addition, you might find putting aside the time to do the exercises easier than if you were in a relationship.

That said, you can still run through the partner exercises purely in your mind. Interestingly, the mind can't tell between real and imagined situations. When you play something in your imagination, your mind and body believes that it is really happening. This brilliant ability of the mind is actually a big part of the problem with vaginismus. The pain we anticipate before penetration is mostly what leads to the pain happening.

So you don't fully believe me about the mind not being able to tell the difference between real and imagined? Have you ever gotten scared from watching a horror movie and remained scared for the rest of the evening despite knowing deep down that you are safe and that vampires/ghosts don't exist?

Have you ever played the game where you imagine a ripe lemon which is full of juice? No? Okay well go ahead, imagine a lemon. Think of its color and texture as you dig your nails into its skin. Think of how it smells when you do that as the citrus scent is released into the air. Now imagine cutting into the lemon and seeing the clear juice spreading underneath. Imagine taking a big juicy slice and biting into it. Really biting in so that the juice squirts all the way to the back of your mouth with its juicy sourness.

Okay, now check your mouth. If you have imagined the lemon as I described (not just read the words but actually imagined those various sensations), then you will notice you have more saliva in your mouth now.

So you have just proved to yourself that your mind cannot tell the difference between real and imagined. So go ahead and imagine doing the exercises with a partner if you wish. And of course the beauty is that you can imagine the exercises going exactly as you would wish with a caring and understanding partner and your body reacting in a more and more relaxed way. Try it out! You could for example add a 5-minute visualization of these partner exercises before you go to bed each night on top of your solo exercises.

8. PART FOUR: SUPPORT, SUPPORTING AND ALTERNATIVE TREATMENTS

Vaginismus is highly varied from one individual to the next in its causes and contributing factors. Therefore, you may or may not be offered other treatment options besides the ones I have already addressed. Health professionals, for example, point out the importance of certain aspects and habits in your daily routine that may affect the health of your pelvic floor muscles. These are:

– Making sure you get adequate rest and sleep. It is during sleep that muscles rest.

– Eating a healthy diet with plenty of fiber to ensure regular bowel movements as constipation can have a negative effect on your pelvic floor muscles.

– Regularly exercising using a routine that includes stretching and relaxing of muscles.

– Supplementing your diet. Talk to your health specialist or a trained naturopath about whether supplementation would be useful for you as there is a link between the health of your muscles and sufficient intake of certain vitamins, minerals and other nutrients. Some, as mentioned in the book *Healing Painful Sex*, include magnesium malate or citrate, vitamin D3, omega 3, and gamma-linolenic acid. However, don't just take these nutrients on a whim as this may not be beneficial for you and at best end up to be a waste of money.

Alternative treatments and options

– In some cases muscle relaxants are prescribed for women who find it difficult to insert a dilator. The muscle relaxant is taken before dilator therapy, sometimes under guidance in the medical professional's practice along with supervised dilator therapy.

– Good results have been obtained in studies that incorporate hypnosis in the treatment plan.

– Medication can be prescribed to lessen feelings of anxiety and depression. I'm uncomfortable with their use for this purpose and recommend you work through your emotions with a therapist instead. People often find they have to face the underlying emotions later anyway – as well as any side effects of coming off the medication. Again, this is a situation where you have to decide what is right for you.

– In the extreme medication realm (in my opinion) is the use of botox. I find this treatment option baffling and the literature I have read on it also warns that in the long term the botoxed muscles can get weaker and lead to further complications down the line.

– And finally, another extreme option for treating vaginismus is surgery. I have heard of this happening, however I have not heard how successful it is in the long term. My reaction to this treatment option is one of criticism, nevertheless, I do respect each person will make decisions that feel right for them. My main concern here is that the psychological component to vaginismus might get ignored.

Ignoring underlying causes of illnesses and treating just the symptoms reminds me of the oil light in my car. You know, the one that turns on when your oil is getting low? Well, I learned that when that light comes on, I need to check the oil level as soon as I can and most likely I'll need to fill up the engine with additional oil.

But what happens if we ignore that light? Well, running a car with low levels of oil means the filter starts to clog and dirty oil circulates the engine, wearing it out far quicker than if it were full. Continue to ignore the light and you cause even more damage as the oil turns to sludge. Ignore it for a long time or pretend the problem doesn't exist and eventually the engine blows and you need to replace it.

Now, we cannot replace our vaginas ladies, and thank goodness nothing will explode down there, but the way I see it, vaginismus is like that little oil light, telling us that something is wrong that needs our attention, not our stubborn ignoring.

How to get support from your partner

We've looked at many things you can do to help yourself to overcome vaginismus, other treatments and approaches to consider as well as the practicalities of how to create an enjoyable sex life with your partner. You may, however, still be wondering how to get your partner involved in your healing journey and how to get them not just involved, but involved in a way that he or she is a useful source of support.

If you have vaginismus and you are in a relationship, including your partner in your healing plan ideally adds another source of support which can be extremely helpful in your treatment. Some steps you can take to increase the likelihood that your partner will be a source of support and not a source of stress are:

1. Address your situation and what you know about vaginismus as honestly and open as you can.

2. Make sure that you let them know you want to work on it and are willing to put the time and effort into working towards a healthy and relaxed sexual relationship with them.

3. Tell them how you think they can help. Ask if they would be willing to do what you would like of them.

4. Let him or her know how it would benefit you both by having them attend any therapy sessions with you.

5. Explain the benefits of sensate focusing exercises and how their joining you helps your mind and body learn how to be relaxed during intimacy and ultimately during sexual intercourse.

6. Listen without judgment when they want to express their frustration, sadness, confusion, etc about you suffering from vaginismus. Most likely, they are not angry or frustrated at you, but at the situation. Accept that this is not easy for them either.

7. Approach it as a team. Let them know that you appreciate their help.

8. In whatever way that you are comfortable, help your partner still get his or her sexual needs met. There is no reason why they should miss out on touch, intimacy and sexual release because of your having vaginismus. Part of this is also being okay with them masturbating and pleasuring themselves. Show them your love throughout your treatment process and work with a therapist on any issues that come up around this topic.

What you can do to support your partner with vaginismus

You might have bought this book because someone you know has vaginismus and you would like to help her or it may be that someone has asked you to read it because they have vaginismus and would like your support. Either way, here are the key factors to being a support as they work through their treatment and the exercises in this book.

Understanding: Take some time to read up on the experience of vaginismus (congratulations, if you are reading this comment, it means you have already started this process). Also, because vaginismus can vary quite dramatically from one woman to the next, talk to your partner and find out what their experience of it is.

Empathy: Put yourself in her shoes and get a feel for what she's going through. Showing empathy with caring comments will help her feel not pressured and able to relax with you sexually down the track – because you understand what is going on for her. In fact, you may be the first person who gives her the feeling of being understood if you do this.

Patience: Working through vaginismus with its physical complications and the underlying emotional elements can take quite some time. Meanwhile, enjoy the things that you easily connect through – such as hobbies, and emotionally connecting by sharing time to talk about dreams together as well as what's on your minds at the end of each day. Touch in ways that work for you both and if there is a time when she feels uncomfortable and wants to stop, then stop!

Take it into your own hands: For your partner, vaginismus might lead to a hugely frustrating situation of her wanting to be able to have sex with you and her body just not letting her. In this case, there is no end to other sexual experiences you can share together and of course she can help you reach climax without vaginal intercourse, in the same way that you can help her also have an orgasm through non-penetrative ways. Additionally, you can 'give each other a hand' as you each bring yourselves to climax. However, when you work through the sensate exercises over a period of time, you will forgo sexual contact for that time.

As your partner works through the steps in this book and any therapy or additional treatment, there might also be times where she asks that you stop touching her at that specific time or generally wants to avoid touch for a while. If that happens, look after your own needs. And by that I don't mean go off and have an affair. I mean masturbate. Again, you will find out if your partner is comfortable to join you as you do so or not.

Some people find it too hard to stay in a relationship where sexual intercourse is not possible and whether you are or are not able to do so yourself will depend on many things including your own sex drive and sexual preferences, religious upbringing and rules of the society you live in as well as the depth of your patience and your own emotional response.

Consider getting support for yourself as well: Vaginismus can bring up feelings and emotional issues for partners such as feeling not good enough. It may make you question your attractiveness or sexual ability. It may make you feel uncomfortable about your appearance, or you may feel rejected, sexually frustrated and angry or confused and sad. As with any conflict or challenge in a relationship, it can be a great help to get some professional advice and support so that instead of complicating matters any further for your partner and yourself, you're actually improving your relationship and helping your partner overcome vaginismus.

Giving time: Your partner will need uninterrupted time by herself to complete the exercises in this book. You can be a great support by giving her this time – and leaving her to it; letting her know that you are there for her if she needs you. In addition, there are some tasks in this book that are designed to be done with a partner. Making yourself available to share these experiences is not only a great way to actively support your partner, but you might be pleasantly surprised at how your relationship and your connection with each other is deepened. The safety of having task boundaries also offers an increased chance that your partner feels able to explore some activities that may not have worked in the past.

Encouragement: I understand that if you find your partner sexually attractive and have a healthy sex drive yourself, that you might be rearing to have sex with her. While you can't solve vaginismus for your partner or push her to 'sort it out' as such, what you can do is gently encourage her to take whatever steps are required in order to keep on track. And that might include not having sex for a while.

For starters you can encourage her to feel safe to talk about the topic with you by listening and taking the time to try to understand and show love regardless. Secondly, you can encourage her to read not only this book but perhaps other books, articles and self-help techniques. Thirdly, for some women, taking this healing journey without professional support is near impossible. Help her find a good therapist that she feels comfortable with and support her to talk about vaginismus with her doctor or gynecologist. Some women's doctors naturally find out that something is wrong when they attempt an examination or pap-smear. For other women, only they and their partners know something isn't right due to their inability to have sexual intercourse or the woman's pain during it. That said, she may want to work through this issue herself and it is her choice to do so. Insisting she get professional help in this case may just cause extra friction. An ongoing discussion of her progress would be better.

What you can do to support your daughter with vaginismus

First of all, it has to be said, if you have the kind of relationship with your daughter in which she feels comfortable telling you about something like this, then well done! You have obviously built up a lot of trust through your actions, honesty and openness around the topic of sex and sexuality and in general.

However, it is nevertheless important that you respect that she has shared this highly personal and maybe scary or embarrassing experience with you. If she's still young, then your reaction will affect her sex life and relationships for the rest of her life. So tread gently. Gently and with love.

Do not make judgmental comments about her being too young to be having sex – now is not the time for that talk. Nor is it appropriate to probe into her sex life or ask unnecessary questions.

Show kindness and normalize the situation. What do I mean by that? Well she's possibly freaking out inside and the last thing she needs is for you to start freaking out as well. So make neutral comments, for example that it can happen sometimes and for a number of reasons. Point out to her that just because she has it now, it doesn't mean she will always have it. That it can be treated and that most women overcome vaginismus.

Ask her if she has thought of talking to someone about it like a therapist or doctor who knows more than you might and who has a neutral viewpoint (in comparison to someone they know). Depending on her answer, you can ask if she would like you to help her find someone and if she would like you or someone else to accompany her or if she wants to go alone.

What you can do to support your friend with vaginismus

Listen and don't try to fix the problem by offering unasked for advice. Just be there for them and allow them to tell you about what's going on for them. Show respect for their honesty and the fact that they are sharing this with you. It's not necessarily an easy thing to share and definitely something for you to keep confidential. Ask if there is anything you can do to help.

For friends, family and others – What to say and what not to say

Examples of what not to say:
It's just because you're a virgin. It's probably just your hymen that needs to be broken.
You just need to push harder.
Chill out, you just need to relax.
Oh my god, have you been raped?? I heard about there being a connection between that and this!
Stop overreacting, you just need to use more lube.
Why are you clenching your muscles like that? Don't you like me!?
You've never been comfortable with intimacy.
You're always so closed off.
You're just making it up.

What you could say instead:
Would you like to talk about it?
Would you like to see someone to get help – like a doctor?
Is there anything you would like me to do to help?
(Yes, it's really that simple!)

In my case, I was still very young when I had vaginismus. The thought didn't occur to either myself or my boyfriend to seek professional help. All we knew was that it was highly frustrating and draining for us both. We didn't know anything about vaginismus and had never heard of it happening to anyone else. We didn't have any logical answers and thus all we knew was that sexual intercourse just didn't work for us no matter how hard we tried.

I didn't have access to the internet back then, and I'm pretty sure that even if I did, the wealth of knowledge that exists and is so easily accessible today just wasn't online then. So we couldn't just search online for 'painful sex' which is what I am sure I would do now if I were in the same situation today. On top of that, although I read several books on sex, none of them referred to this condition. We ended up coming to our own conclusions out of ignorance. He figured that I just didn't want sex or was scared of him or that I was afraid of intimacy, whereas I concluded that it was a combination of still being a virgin and his penis being too big for me.

The fact however was, that he was the first male that I had been sexually intimate with at that point in my life. Thus I was hardly qualified to make an educated judgment about his size, because I had very little previous experience to draw on – but that didn't enter my mind at that stage. My theory and the reason why I kept trying was that it *should* be possible. He had had sex with other girls before and it had worked for them, so it had to work for me too. My alternative belief was that we somehow just didn't physically match and there was nothing we could do about it. I didn't really want to accept that as an option. But it seemed there was little other choice. Oh, how I wanted the information back then that is available today!

Tips on choosing your health professionals: Such as gynecologist, sex therapist, health practitioner and doctor

This is an important topic, because some people put up with vaginismus for their whole life without seeking professional help. While it is absolutely your choice to do so, it saddens me to think that those women miss out on this aspect of their sexuality and face the negative effects that their pain as well as their physical and emotional discomfort have in relationships, to their self-esteem, body image and so forth.

In this book I keep referring to the two elements present in vaginismus: the psychological/emotional component and the physical/muscular reaction. In an ideal world, women would get support and guidance to address both. It is your choice and often people like to see if they can solve a problem themselves before getting help. I totally understand that because that is how I typically approach things myself. That is also why I have included all of the exercises in this book. However, some people will enjoy and greatly benefit from having extra support along their journey.

And thus ... the key factors to consider when choosing your professionals are:

1. Check they are qualified and belong to a professional organization.

2. Gauge your gut reaction in the first meeting or correspondence. Do you feel comfortable discussing the situation with them?

3. Most importantly, do they listen and take you seriously? Far too many women are told their vaginas are healthy, and nothing is wrong with them, while the women know that clearly something is not right.

4. How long have they been practicing?

5. Have they worked with this condition before?

6. This is a personal preference but something you might also want to consider: Do they actually have a plan and techniques to help you solve this? There are many different types of therapies, some of which create clear plans and others which do not.

For example, clients come to me for all sorts of issues. Often they come after working with someone for months or even years where they just talk about their problem and drag up the past, but don't actually do anything to move forward by identifying solutions and taking action towards their goals. These sessions can be as emotionally draining as the problem itself. I have also experienced this kind of therapy style myself and prefer the kind that has a clear focus on getting results. Due to this, you may consider looking for someone trained in modalities such as solution-focused counseling, Neuro Linguistic Programming (NLP), Cognitive Behavioral Therapy

(CBT) or hypnotherapy as part of their training background. I'm pointing out those particular ones because they are either the ones that have good results in studies or have worked for me and that's why I trained in them. But have a look around at what's available and find a therapy modality that clicks with you.

These are just some ideas, mainly coming from my own experiences as a client as well as working as a therapist myself and knowing from that viewpoint what I look for in health professionals if I require them.

9. PART FIVE: IN CONCLUSION - THE ENDING TO MY VAGINISMUS STORY

I have told you numerous times in this book that you have to do what feels right for you. In my case, when I think about it now, not going to the doctor and getting diagnosed when I had vaginismus in my youth turned out alright in the end.

As it happened, after much discussion with a close friend, I ended up putting most of the blame on my first boyfriend's penis size. I remember talking with my friend about it and her agreeing with me as I asked in exasperation "what else could it be?" We knew that it couldn't be my hymen by then. So it had to be that we didn't physically match; a serious case of bad luck. Or so we thought. And my teenage theory seemed to be proved correct with the next guy I had sex with. His penis was significantly smaller (at least enough that I consciously took note). And it was as if my unconscious mind seeing a smaller penis allowed my muscles to relax fully, making intercourse possible and in that instant breaking the anxiety-pain feedback loop. I never had any physical difficulties from that day on. Seriously.

So, that leaves a question that you might be wondering about and one that was certainly on my mind after having sex. Was my first boyfriend really too big for me? Were we a mismatch after all? Well, we already know that the vagina is a wonderfully stretchy part of our body which should make this question redundant, especially as we cannot put the pain down to him being too far inside me and hitting the cervix, right? Well, a number of years later I got to test my theory during a time when I was single. We decided to try again.

My memory from that day is one of thinking he still felt very 'big' for me, but intercourse was possible with him. This allowed me to finally put that question to rest. At the time, I still didn't understand why it hadn't worked at all back when we were younger. However, I concluded at the time that if we ever got back together (that day turned out to be a one-off), it would have simply been necessary to spend more time on my arousal and explore various sex positions to identify those that worked for us both.

I now hear some of you asking, "Yes but why did it work then and not earlier?" To answer this, I think it is relevant to understand the type of relationship I had with the boyfriend who was my second sexual partner. My relationship with him had felt quite controlled. He often attempted to control my behavior and limit activities which he did not approve of. Contact with my first boyfriend was also made forbidden. I remember when I finally broke free from that second relationship that I felt wonderfully in control of my life again and my freedom to choose.

Going 'all the way' with my first boyfriend was one way I was able to express this freedom of choice and my individuality. In addition, remember I'd thought our difficulties had been due to his size or my virginity or a combination of both. Having by then well and truly lost my virginity, I assumed that it would no longer hinder us and it turned out that the size in itself no longer was that big of a deal either.

So what about other psychological aspects that contributed to my experience of vaginismus? What else could have caused it and what allowed that physical muscle-clenching to disappear the way it did?

My conclusion after working on my issues and during further research of vaginismus, is that the cause behind vaginismus for me could have been due to quite a number of elements. Looked at individually, none of them stands out as an obvious cause, and none by itself is enough to have caused it (otherwise many more women would experience vaginismus). The role that each played in contributing to my experience is really anyone's guess and there is no way of really knowing. That said, I had the following combination of *possible* contributing factors:

– A Catholic education and the accompanying fear-mongering about sexually transmitted diseases, teen pregnancies and graphic birth videos.

– A sexual partner who I didn't fully trust - he had a reputation of being promiscuous. Perhaps, as a result, unconsciously I didn't feel comfortable sharing that level of intimacy with him. I say unconsciously, because consciously I desperately wanted it to work.

– Fear and anxiety that losing my virginity was going to be extremely painful and embarrassing.

– His penis was on the wide end of the scale. Our first attempt were painful so we stopped, leading to future expectation of pain combined with a fantastic imagination setting up quite an intense fear-pain cycle.

– Right at the start of one of our early attempts, the condom broke. This freaked me out because I had learned at school that you could get pregnant from pre-ejaculation fluid. Full of embarrassment and discomfort, we went to a family planning center the next day and got the emergency contraceptive pill. I was too scared for a while to try to have sex again for fear that the condom would break again. After that incident – my first boyfriend told me many years later that – he could feel me tensing each time we tried. This is something I wasn't aware of at the time, which really highlights how unconscious the physical reaction of vaginismus can be.

– A childhood upbringing with a general awkwardness

around the topic of sex – my sex education was severely lacking.

– The sense that I was old enough and needed to get the "deed" done which added more and more pressure and stress with each failed attempt.

– An apprehension that I wouldn't find a boyfriend who loved me. Nor one who I loved and would feel comfortable enough to share that level of intimacy with.

– The situation wasn't helped by my boyfriend having to leave the bed to sleep away from me in case his parents walked in, which lead to me being alone while still tearful after each attempt. He wasn't a complete jerk though – he would try to comfort me, but I was inconsolable and he would eventually give up and go to his bed feeling dejected himself.

Had it gone differently and I had sought medical advice, I may have been given the vaginismus diagnosis. I may have been prescribed anti-anxiety medication, and I may have become convinced that something was seriously wrong with me after all. From my work with clients, I have seen firsthand how labels and diagnoses can stick in the mind and have a negative psychological effect for years. Diagnoses often influence what a person believes is possible for them or not. Therefore a big part of a person's journey is sometimes learning to see themselves as something other than their condition.

I consider myself extremely fortunate that the vaginismus

went away without any conscious effort, but if it had continued with my second boyfriend I would have needed to treat it in some way – either by finding a self-help approach that I could follow like this book, or by seeing a doctor. The main point of what I'm saying to you now is not to allow it to take over your life and prevent you from having the kind of relationship you want.

So, ultimately, my advice is to trust your gut on this one. Only you will be able to figure out what the right treatment path is for you and what you need in your individual situation.

Further realizations

I attended a meditation training before I started dating my second boyfriend. I had started to regularly meditate and use guided visualizations to relax as well as for spiritual exploration. It's possible my new skills in accessing a relaxed space and calming any anxious thoughts had a positive spin-off for my subsequent sex life. Maybe. It's all speculation really. There is no way to get a computer printout on what made the most difference or which of these aspects were the most important pieces in the puzzle.

It's also important to point out that although I could physically have sex with my second boyfriend, I still had many issues and challenges with sex, body image, sexuality and confidence. I had to overcome them before

I could start to completely embrace all aspects of myself and relax enough to really get the deep connection and fun sexual experiences that I had wanted all along. This is where therapeutic support became a really important part of my healing story and it took quite a number of years to find a therapy style that I liked and then to work through all the different issues that came up. That said, I'm not unrealistic enough to think that my sex life will always be as fantastic as it is now. I know I have interesting life changes ahead of me including menopause and other age related stages. Of course if I choose to have children, then that too will affect my sex life.

In any case, I will take the same approach that whatever I might face, someone out there will have written a book about it or included information in a book. I know I can talk about issues with my husband and a couple of close friends who I trust. I can also work through issues with the self-help tools I have picked up over the years in my own discoveries and from my professional training. And if I still can't solve it, I can go see a professional to get some external guidance.

I truly believe that there is a solution to everything so long as you are willing to learn new techniques, embrace new ideas, and open to challenging and ultimately changing any beliefs that limit you in your life.

I would love to hear about your journey and what has worked for you. I'm also happy for you to contact me with ideas of how I could improve this book or if you have any questions. Also, remember that you can give me a review online where you purchased this ebook. I'm sure other women will appreciate your honest opinion!

My email address is: maree@nwow.co.nz and my website is: www.nwow.co.nz.

I wish you all the best in your journey! And I hope that this book can contribute to you getting the comfortable and enjoyable sexual experiences that you want in your life.

Warm regards,

Maree Stachel-Williamson

10. RECOMMENDED READING

If you are interested in further reading you can have a look through the reference list where I have listed the books, articles and websites I have have taken information from for this book. There are four that really stood out for me and are well worth the read:

www.vaginismus.com. This is a great website and information resource. I imagine you'll find answers to any further questions you have about vaginismus that I haven't addressed here.

Healing painful sex: A woman's guide to confronting, diagnosing, and treating sexual pain. This book by Deborah Coady and Nancy Fish details the wide variety of treatments available. It also covers the many different types and causes of pain during sex which might be useful for those who experience one of the other painful sex conditions in addition to or instead of vaginismus. Strangely, the authors don't like the word vaginismus and try to argue that it is outdated. They prefer the general term vestibulodynia, but I think they are misguided as the definition of vaginismus is restricted to the muscle-clenching experience whereas vestibulodynia is a very general term. Calling vaginismus vestibulodynia just confuses the matter in my opinion. Keep this in mind if you read the book.

Sex life: How our sexual experiences define who we are. Written by Dr. Pamela Stephenson-Connolly. This was such an interesting read because the author follows the experience of sexuality from birth to old age. With a refreshingly open writing style, this is a book I highly recommend if you are wondering what is 'normal' when it comes to sex.

The heart of desire: Keys to the pleasures of love – by Stella Resnick. This is a really comprehensive book for anyone wanting to read about how to have a pleasurable sex life, but also how to keep sexual desire alive over a long period of time within a relationship. The author includes her viewpoint as a psychologist as well as the latest scientific research and findings from neuroscience.

11. GLOSSARY

Clitoris: An organ which exists purely for pleasure. Often thought of as only the small 'bulb' at the top of the vulva, the clitoris extends deep within the vagina as well as along the labia.

Dyspareunia: The general medical term used for painful intercourse or sexual pain. The intensity of pain varies from person to person, and can range from mild pain during sex which is only noticed afterward, to the pain preventing sex altogether.

Labia majora: Part of the vulva – the two outer 'lips', covered by pubic hair in adults (unless otherwise removed).

Labia minora: Part of the vulva – the two inner 'lips' that directly surround the vaginal opening and urethra. The word 'minora' and the implication that they are 'minor' compared to the labia majora can be confusing for some women as the size and shape varies widely from hanging low past the labia majora or only 'poking out' a little.

Libido: Interest in sex. When referring to someone having a low or high libido (or sex drive as it is sometimes called), it means they have little or a lot of interest in sex respectively. Many things can affect a person's libido including stress levels, medications and hormonal changes.

Sexual arousal: The awakening of sexual desire which results in physiological and psychologically changes in the body as it prepares for sexual activity. In the female body, some of these changes among many are: erection of nipples and clitoris, swelling and darkening of labia, vaginal lubrication, pupils becoming dilated, increase in breathing and heart rate.

Vagina: A muscular and elastic 3-5 inch long internal passage from uterus to vulva. Some people mistakenly call the external genitalia (vulva) the vagina as well.

Vaginitis: Painful sex due to infection which may be resulting from sexually transmitted diseases or due to a yeast infection.

Vaginismus: Painful and/or impossible sex and penetration due to the clenching of the pelvic floor muscles. Muscle tension can be so intense as to restrict penetration of any kind. In this case, it can feel as though you are hitting a wall. A less but still painful version of vaginismus is when the muscles partially contracts allowing restricted penetration. In this case, penetration is possible but still results in pain and discomfort.

Vestibulodynia: Pain upon touch at the vestibule – the area where the vulva meets the opening to the vagina. Soreness and tenderness can be upon vaginal penetration or even through light touch. The amount of pain varies from woman to woman. Some are able to have penetrative sex with a small amount of discomfort; for others even light touch to the area creates pain. Continuing penetration despite pain can lead to pelvic floor muscles clenching as a stress response and vaginismus.

Vulva: The external female genitalia. In other words, what you can see from the outside in contrast to the internal workings which you see in biology diagrams.

Vulvodynia: Pain from a burning sensation in the vulva area due to irritation or hypersensitivity in the nerve fibers in the vulval skin. Pain can also occur without being touched or during penetration. The pain experienced is not due to any infection or skin condition.

12. REFERENCES

Abramov, L.A. (1976). Sexual life and sexual frigidity among women developing acute myocardial infarction. *Journal of Biobehavioural Medicine. Psychosomatic Medicine, 38*(6),418-425.

American Psychiatric Association. (n.d.). *Highlights of changes from DSM-IV-TR to DSM-5.* Retrieved September 5, 2013, from www.psychiatry.org/File %20Library/Practice/DSM/DSM-5/Changes-from-DSM-IV-TR--to-DSM-5.pdf

Anonymous. (2013, June). 100 days of sex. *Australian Men's Health.* 78 – 83.

Bortz II, W.M., & Stickrod, R. (2010). *The roadmap to 100: The breakthrough science of living a long and healthy life.* New York, United States: Palgrave Macmillan.

Braverman, E.R., & Capria, E. (2011) *Younger sexier you: Look and feel 15 years younger by having the best sex of your life*. New York, United States: Rodale Inc.

Castleman, M. (2011, March 1). The hymen: A membrane widely misunderstood. The truth behind all those bloody sheets. [Web log post]. Retrieved from http://www.psychologytoday.com/blog/all-about-sex/201103/the-hymen-membrane-widely-misunderstood

Chia, M., & Carlton Abrams, R. (2005). *The multi-orgasmic woman: sexual secrets every woman should know*. London, England: Rodale International Ltd.

Coady, D., & Fish, N. (2011) *Healing painful sex: A woman's guide to confronting, diagnosing, and treating sexual pain*. Berkeley, California, United States: Seal Press.

Davidson, T., & Key, K. (2012). Vaginismus. In Kristin Key (Ed.), *The Gale Encyclopedia of Mental Health*. 2 Vols. (3rd ed). Detroit, United States: Gale.

Doyle, M. (1998). *Woman's body: An owners manual*. Hertfordshire, UK: Wordsworth Editions Ltd.

Hartman, D. (2010). Therapy of vaginismus by hypnotic desensitization. *Journal of Heart Centered Therapies*, *13*(1), 107(1).

Kellogg Spadt, S., Iorio, J., Yonaitis Fariello, J., & Whitmore, K.E. (2012). Vaginal dilation: When it's indicated and tips on teaching it. *OBG Management*, *24*(12)

Komisaruk, B.R., Beyer-Flores, C., & Whipple, B. (2006) *The science of orgasm*. (1st ed.). Baltimore, United States: Johns Hopkins University Press.

Kuchinskas, S. (2009). *The chemistry of connection: How the oxytocin response can help you find trust, intimacy, and love*. Oakland, Canada: New Harbinger Publications.

Masters, W.H., Johnson, V.E., & Kolodny, R.C. (1986). *Master and Johnson on sex and human loving*. Boston, United States: Little, Brown and Company Inc.

melodiousmsm. (2011, November 30). The internal clitoris. [Web log post]. Retrieved from http://blog.museumofsex.com/the-internal-clitoris/

Ploog, K.. (1999). *Voicecoaching: Das trainingskonzept fuer gesangstechnik*. Bonn, Germany: Voggenreiter Verlag

Resnick, S. (2012). *The heart of desire: Keys to the pleasures of love*. New Jersey, United States: John Wiley & Sons, Inc.

Stephenson-Connolly, P. (2011). *Sex life: How our sexual experiences define who we are*. London, England: Vermilion.

Stuart, B. (2010). The relative health benefits of different sexual activities. *The Journal of Sexual Medicine*. 7(4pt1), 1336-1361

Vaginismus.com: Helping women overcome sexual pain. Retrieved September 15, 2013, from http://www.vaginismus.com

Vulval Pain Society. (2013). Retrieved September 23, 2013, from http://www.vulvalpainsociety.org

Wade, J. (2004). *Transcendent sex: When lovemaking opens the veil*. New York, United States: Paraview Pocket

Books.

Weed, S.S. (2011). *Down there: Sexual and reproductive health. The wise woman way*. New York, United States: Ash Tree Publishing.

Westheimer, R., Grunebaum, A. & Lehu, P. (2012). *Sexually speaking: What every woman needs to know about sexual health*. New Jersey, United States: John Wiley & Sons, Inc.

Whipple, B., & Komisaruk, B.R. (1985). Elevation of pain threshold by vaginal stimulation in women. *Pain, 21*(4), 357-367

Whipple, B., Richards, E., Tepper, M., & Komisaruk, B.R. (1996). Sexual response in women with complete spinal cord injury. *Sexuality and Disability, 14*(3), 191-201.

ABOUT THE AUTHOR

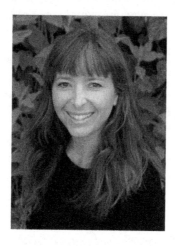

Maree Stachel-Williamson is a therapist who incorporates her own life experiences with professional knowledge from her work and the latest research and experts' perspectives.

Honest and to the point, Maree shares her expertise with the aim of empowering people to find solutions that work for them.

Maree has a diverse training background which includes NLP (Neuro-Linguistic Programming), Person-Centered Counseling, EFT (Emotional Freedom Techniques), Family and Structural Constellation Work, Ericksonian and Clinical Hypnotherapy, Time-Line Therapy ™, Clean Language and TFH Kinesiology (Touch for Health).

Other e-books written by Maree available for purchase:

- Female Masturbation: Simple Pleasures to Mind-Blowing Orgasms
- The Baby Dilemma: How to Decide

www.nwow.co.nz

Made in the USA
Las Vegas, NV
30 January 2023

66523057R00069